BEYOND VALIUM

Beyond Valium

*The Brave New World of
Psychochemistry*

Seymour Rosenblatt, M.D.
and
Reynolds Dodson

G. P. Putnam's Sons
New York

The author gratefully acknowledges permission to quote from the following
sources:
  From Sad to Glad, Nathan S. Kline, MD.
    Copyright © 1974 by Nathan S. Kline.
    Reprinted by permission of Julian Bach Literary Agency, Inc.
  Drug Treatment of Medical Disorders, "Recent Genetic and Biochemical
      Approaches to Schizophrenia," Seymour S. Kety.
    Copyright © 1976 by Raven Press.
    Reprinted by permission of Raven Press.
  British Medical Journal, "Drug Lag Bad: Drug Lack Worse."
    Copyright © 1980 by the *British Medical Journal*.
    Reprinted by permission of the *British Medical Journal*.
  Journal of Projective Techniques and Personality Assessment,
    "Psychological Variables in Human Cancer," B. Klopfer.
    Copyright © 1957 by the J.P.T.P.A.
    Reprinted by permission of the J.P.T.P.A.

Library of Congress Cataloging in Publication Data

Rosenblatt, Seymour.
  Beyond valium.

  Includes index.
  1. Psychopharmacology. I. Dodson, Reynolds.
II. Title. [DNLM: 1. Diazepam—Popular works.
2. Mental disorders—Drugs therapy—Popular works.
QV 77.9 R813b]
RC483.R6 1981   615'.78   81-2381
ISBN 0-399-12577-9   AACR2

PRINTED IN THE UNITED STATES OF AMERICA

Acknowledgments

For their considerable support and hospitality, I would like to thank Dr. Rosenblatt's staff, particularly Barbara Berman and Georgette Ruta, who endured so many interruptions and inconveniences. For the historical material on Valium, we owe additional thanks to Al Zobel and Bob Jones of Roche. For her emotional support (and considerable pharmaceutical knowledge), I am indebted to my dearest friend, Susan Roessner of Botto, Roessner, Horne & Messinger. Last but not least, a posthumous thanks to the ill-starred soul whose life and death helped spur my curiosity.

Reynolds Dodson
New York City
January 1981

Contents

Introduction

Within siren's cry of Mt. Sinai Hospital, facing Central Park across Fifth Avenue, an unmarked door leads onto the sidewalk in front of what appears to be a fashionable apartment building. There is no shingle outside, no plaque saying Doctor's Office. The entrance is designed for anonymity. Anyone using the buzzer on this door might be calling on a friend or making a delivery.

How I came to push that buzzer is, even in retrospect, an untidy story. It involved a friend who had been suffering from depression and who later took his life with alcohol and barbiturates. Previously he had been taking antidepressants—tricyclics and MAO inhibitors. They failed to save him. Probably nothing could have saved him. There are some people, unfortunately, who are beyond salvation.

My friend's adventures into these therapies had left me curious. What were these drugs, and how did they help people? I was particularly surprised to learn that MAO inhibitors could create a cerebral hemorrhage when consumed with pickled herring.

Armed with an assignment from a national magazine, I set out to do research on drugs and psychiatry. I wanted to know what had become of Dr. Freud and to find out what these pills might do to people. Clearly psychiatry had taken a sharp turn somewhere, and just as clearly, the public was unaware of it. Like everyone, I had heard of Valium, but I had no idea of the dimensions of the story behind it.

During the course of this research, one of the doctors I interviewed was Seymour Rosenblatt of Mt. Sinai Hospital. He was a professor of psychiatry at Mt. Sinai's College of Medicine and chief of that institution's Affective Disorders and Lithium Clinic. This was how I came to the unmarked door. It was the entrance to Sy Rosenblatt's private offices. When I left two hours later, my mind was racing. I knew that I had uncovered the tip of an iceberg.

A few weeks later I called Dr. Rosenblatt. "Would you be interested in doing a book?" I asked. "A science book, written in idiomatic language, that would explain the principles of drugs and brain chemistry?"

After a moment's hesitation he said he would. "I think it might be of service," he said. We met again. A deal was struck. He would be the voice, I would be his typewriter.

In the year that followed certain events took place that gave added urgency to the subject of this book. Newspapers began jumping on the Valium bandwagon, running series about prescriptive-drug abuse. There was a Senate investigation in Washington. Psychiatry and drugs made the covers of *Time* and *Newsweek*. Publishers also joined the fray with books like *The Tranquilizing of America* and *I'm Dancing as Fast as I Can*.

Meanwhile I was up to my neck in science, trying to master the vocabulary of both the chemist and the analyst. Patiently, methodically, Sy Rosenblatt would explain. Doggedly, simplistically, I would assist in the translation.

Several problems presented themselves immediately. One was inherent in the title of the book. To the chemist Valium is not very significant. It is not in the same league with chlorpromazine or lithium. In the end, however, we both agreed that the use of Valium was a significant social phenomenon. With apologies to

10

Roche Laboratories, we chose it as a focal point, since it is the mood-changing substance with which most people have had experience.

Another problem—mine more than his—was the inclusion of Sy Rosenblatt's own contributions. I would have liked to have elaborated his personal triumphs, which, as I have learned from his associates, are indeed considerable. He is one of the most respected psychopharmacologists in America, not only as a researcher but as a practicing healer. A "doctor's doctor," he spends much of his day advising fellow psychiatrists and handling referrals.

My inability to mythologize his accomplishments is not a sign of his false modesty. It is truly a reflection of this physician's personality. He is a scientist and a healer, not a self-promoter. Most of what I learned about him came from others. He was a pioneer in the biology of electroshock. He is a frequent adviser to the pharmaceutical industry in the fields of education, drug therapy and drug safety.

Perhaps the greatest testimony comes from Mt. Sinai itself, where he teaches at the Page and William Black School of Medicine. For years he has been considered one of the few psychopharmacologists who is qualified to lecture on his specialty to other doctors.

These obstacles notwithstanding, the many months that went into the research of this book have been among the most rewarding in my life. I entered with strong skepticism about psychiatry, the people who practice it and the employment of drugs to relieve psychic agony. I came out with a newfound respect not only for psychopharmacology but for the life sciences in general.

I hope that the reader will share some of my enthusiasm.

Reynolds Dodson
New York City
January 1981

It is only by means of the sciences of life that the quality of life can be radically changed. The release of atomic energy marks a great revolution in human history, but . . . the really revolutionary revolution is to be achieved, not in the external world, but in the souls and flesh of human beings.

—Aldous Huxley

In view of the intimate connection between things physical and mental, we may look forward to a day when paths of knowledge will be opened up leading from organic biology and chemistry to the field of neurotic phenomena.

—Sigmund Freud

That humanity at large will ever be able to dispense with Artificial Paradises seems very unlikely.

—Aldous Huxley

BEYOND VALIUM

1

The Mind-Body Connection

In the next twenty years humanity will witness one of the greatest revolutions in the history of medicine. Indeed, in many ways the revolution is already upon us. Television and newspapers worry about "Valiumania"; best-selling books denounce us as a "pill-popping culture"; feminists suggest the existence of a "conspiracy" in which tranquilizers are employed to perpetuate male "control."

As a psychopharmacologist—a "drug doctor," if you will—my life has been touched by much of this controversy. The first important psychoactive drug was discovered at about the time I began my career, and I have spent the last thirty years intimately involved in all phases of psychiatric drug treatment and research. It has been an exciting period. I have watched with satisfaction as countless millions have been released from hellholes of despair. I have seen men and women, their lives in shambles, miraculously rise from the ashes of depression. I have seen schizophrenics learn to communicate sensibly and manic-depressives put away thoughts of suicide. I have seen the emotionally disturbed begin to be treated like humans, admitted to hospitals instead of interned behind gray walls somewhere. It has been one of the most satisfying careers a person could follow.

But there has been a more negative, misunderstood side of my work, too. I have shared the public's alarm about drug abuse. I have watched mildly anxious people turn into addicts. I have seen legitimate drugs become perverted by our culture, turned into holy grails of euphoria which they were never intended to be. And I have felt frustrated. I have seen intelligent reporters, who should know better, spread the most damaging myths about drugs and their function; I have seen the half-baked notions of faddists and junkies become accepted as fact by an uneducated populace.

In view of this criticism and its effect upon my profession, I feel the time has come to set the record straight—to explain to people how drugs really work and the implications they have for the future. This will not be easy, for it is a very complex subject, an issue fraught with prejudice and emotionalism. I feel a little like the man explaining nuclear fission to the people living around Three Mile Island.

The truth is this: Society today stands on the threshold of a brave new world of chemical control—a world that promises both hope and peril, contentment and fear, progress or disaster. That this threshold exists is undeniable. Scientifically we have already crossed over it. We have seen the future, and while it may not work, it looks promising enough that its pursuit has become inevitable.

Basically what this future consists of is the coming together of three disparate elements: our minds (and how we perceive our environment); our bodies; and what we can produce in a laboratory. Our views of each are changing so profoundly that they threaten to throw our perceptions off axis. Perhaps not since Copernicus and Galileo has there been a wave of new thought so threatening to our complacency.

Consider some of the possibilities currently being promoted by serious scientists:

> In the next twenty years, it has been conjectured, we
> will be able to control people's feelings and emotions.

18

Madness will go the way of smallpox, and mental institutions will become as rare as monasteries.

Everyone will get a decent night's sleep. Senility will be arrested by a pill or an injection. Our memories will be extended beyond their present capacities, and both drug addiction and alcoholism will become things of the past.

Sex offenders will be controlled by medication. Our system of penology will be in the purview of chemistry. Steel bars will be replaced by pharmacological agents, leaving criminals to roam free but restricted from harming people.

We will have *jamais vu* drugs that create feelings of novelty and *déjà vu* drugs to breed familiarity. Both boredom and anxiety will be alleviated, and our sex lives will be enhanced and intensified.

Blood cells will be harnessed to become the psychiatrist's allies. They will become like beasts of burden, hauling drugs throughout our bodies. There will be no side effects, no nausea, no liver damage, and dosages will be reduced to fractions of their present levels.

Drugs will be used to slow the metabolism and induce hibernation for prolonged space travel. The aging process will be decelerated, and time, as we know it, will have little significance.

Finally, we shall emerge into a drug-free society in which genetic engineering precludes mental illness. The substances produced by our biochemists will exactly match those endowed to us by nature.

These are some of the possibilities already being discussed in seminars and medical journals. Exciting? Yes. Frightening? Perhaps. It depends on your viewpoint and your definition of progress. Already the first salvos of criticism have been fired, some of them legitimate, some of them not, but many by people who know little about the subject, addressing a confused public that, understandably, knows less. There is an impression that psychiatrists are "pill happy," that drugs, being unnatural, are inherently evil, that even the most benign of tranquilizers can weaken one's will or erode a user's spirit. There is a suspicion of doctors, a suspicion of drug companies, a suspicion of people who use tranquilizers to "cope" and, finally, a suspicion of America itself, whose culture is thought to have created this phenomenon.

Some of the charges are even more specific. Valium, the most popular target, has been charged with everything from creating psychosis to destroying fetuses to being the equivalent of arsenic. There have been reports linking Valium to fatalities. In a later chapter we'll examine those claims. Suffice it for now to say that they are not true, and they serve no useful purpose beyond scaring the wits out of people.

This is not to say that drugs are panaceas or that their widespread use is not a dangerous phenomenon. Indeed, they are dangerous, because people abuse them, and until recently we have had very little real knowledge of them. Betty Ford was right to warn women about pill dependency. Editorialists are correct to deplore the sale of "street drugs." I'll also admit that there are those in my profession who prescribe drugs too frequently and without proper knowledge of them.

Scientifically, however, there is reason for optimism. We're finally beginning to learn what these substances are all about. It is like piecing together a giant jigsaw puzzle, with the mind itself being the picture that emerges. The importance of this knowledge becomes evident when you realize our dependency on drugs—not just the khat and peyote of the primitives, but the nicotine and alcohol so important to our own culture. John Marks, a leading British scientist, reminds us that mood alteration is a part of many activities, from the compulsive need to complete a crossword puzzle to the willingness to kill ourselves through morphine and heroin addiction. The only difference is the balance of risks and the acceptability of those risks to the society in which we live. But this must not undermine our quest for knowledge and the instinctive need to make life more tolerable.

That we are fulfilling this need, and at a dramatic rate, while enlarging what might be called the doors of our consciousness, is evident in the statistics of the past thirty years, since the first big breakthrough in pharmaceutical therapy.

In 1950, before the advent of psychoactive drugs, our state and county mental hospitals were filled to overflowing. We had 512,501 patients locked behind bars on a full-time basis. By 1975 this number had dropped to 193,436. That's a net reduction of about 62 percent, despite the increase in our population.

Within the same period deaths in those hospitals dropped from 41,280 to 13,401—a reduction of almost 67 percent. What makes these figures even more dramatic is that admissions were up almost two and a half times—from 152,286 to 376,156. This indicates that more people were being reached, if only on a short-term or revolving-door basis. This wouldn't have been possible without drug therapy, and certainly not through traditional analysis.

Simultaneously we are in the process of correcting our excesses, particularly in our usage of the so-called minor tranquilizers. We have seen a dramatic drop-off in both prescription rates and refills of these drugs, including Valium and Librium. According to Dr. Mitchell Balter, dean of statistics for the National Institute of Mental Health, overall sales of Valium-like substances have fallen almost 40 percent since the early seventies. Roche Laboratories, which produces Valium, reports a similar decline in the sale of their product—from a 1975 high of 61.3 million prescriptions to a 1979 low of 38.5 million.

This indicates a healthy trend—and perhaps an anticipatory response to the recent criticism. In other words, by the time the media got around to worrying about it, the tranquilizer fad had already subsided.

Yet mood-changing drugs and our increased understanding of them are having a profound impact on the entire field of medicine. They are bringing the behavioral sciences into the fold of the physical, and they are raising questions of the spirit among the most sawdust-dry anatomists. In the 1940s, when I was in medical school, people were considered to have two sides: There was the physical, which belonged in the realm of the "life sciences," and the mental, which was carved up among various other disciplines.

21

The body, consisting of organs and tissues, was ruled by an unknowable despot called the brain. The brain answered only to one's environment and upbringing—as if it had read Freud and, therefore, existed.

Today we know that the mind and body are interlocked in an inseparable matrix; that all of our thoughts, our perceptions of things, are intimately determined by our chemistry and our nervous system. Indeed, in some ways the body rules the mind. It is the first receptor of everything we experience. Our physiological reactions can color our perceptions—just as what we think, in turn, can alter our bodily functions.

The implications of this interplay are beginning to unravel three thousand years of thought. No longer does it make sense to talk of "duality," as if a person's mind were the master and the body the mere handservant. For doctors and therapists, the medical and the emotional have been fused together. If Freud must be subjected to Hippocrates, so Hippocrates can no longer neglect mankind's spiritual side.

Statistics are already reflecting this shift. Thirty years ago psychiatry was viewed as an art form. Thousands of medical students, not keen on science, went into psychiatry as a way of "helping people." Today this enrollment has dropped precipitously—down 70 percent since 1970. Less than 4 percent of today's medical students will choose psychiatry as their field of specialty. As a result, we now face a psychiatrist shortage. Next year, in county and state medical hospitals, some nine thousand staff positions will go unfilled, despite continued reductions in bed requirements.

Dr. Edward Joseph, a colleague of mine and director of education in Mt. Sinai's Department of Psychiatry, lists some possible causes for this radical shift, all of them stemming from the mind-body revolution. The first is that in the majority of medical schools, science requirements have stiffened considerably. No longer is psychiatry an attractive choice for students who are not interested in biochemistry.

The second is the growth of family medicine as a specialty. For doctors who "like people" this is an appealing alternative. Thirty

22

years ago, when Freud was king, only psychiatry had this humanistic dimension.

Last, psychiatry, is not a money-making field. This may seem surprising in view of the fees that are charged, but despite the notion that it caters to the affluent, it is one of the lowest-paid specialties in the medical profession.

Drug therapy is both the cause and the result of these changes. Without drug therapy we would still have "insane asylums." We would still have thousands of frustrated psychiatrists trying to work miracles by dealing with people's "guilt feelings." We would still be ignorant about the brain and nervous system, because we would not have the incentive to find out more about them. We would be spending longer sessions with fewer patients, and we would still be considered to possess mystical knowledge.

Instead, psychiatry today has become less and less arcane. Having strayed from the enticing abstractions of Freud, we find ourselves in a molecular universe as rigorous yet accessible as astronomy or physics. In some ways I fear that we may have gone too far in this direction. In later chapters I'll return to this point, because I think there are valuable psychoanalytic concepts that are in danger of becoming lost in all the chemical wizardry. But for now our world has become the world of the microscope. It is a world of new words like *enkephalin* and *endorphins*. It is a world where researchers play medical detective, looking for the causes of our misery in our brain cells and in our chemistry.

Ironically, Freud foresaw this. Again and again throughout his life and in his writings, he predicted that the methods he had so meticulously constructed would be eroded and surpassed by advances in biochemistry. Psychoanalysis was always an inefficient process. It was too complex, too time consuming to reach large numbers of people. Freud himself advocated "intense analysis," which in today's economy is largely unaffordable.

This book presents a bag of mixed blessings. It is not to be taken as a road to Utopia, but neither is it to be seen as a blueprint for destruction or the materialization of a Huxleian nightmare. In fact, it might be argued that we have reached a point where we are in a race against ourselves for our own survival. Our destructive

23

capabilities have become so cataclysmic that unless we are willing to change ourselves, we may embrace extinction. The *means* of this change is the point of controversy. There are hundreds of interest groups trying to play God with our future—from moralists to theologians to politicians to army officers, all trying to lay claim to our salvation and our betterment.

Science represents only one such interest group. It argues that the ultimate change must be in people. Neither our environment nor our technology nor our good intentions can save us from destruction, given the frailty of our temperament. This frailty in part is the result of our chemistry. Change our chemistry, and you can assure our survival. Only through such a radical expedient can we guard ourselves against mayhem and holocaust.

So science argues—but is science correct? In the end it is society that will be the judge. We are on the brink of a life-science revolution, and the enormity of that event must not be underestimated. I myself have a number of doubts. I worry about the zealotry I sometimes see in my profession. I am not sure that in our desire to save humanity from destruction, we may not turn people into something that is not quite so worth saving. You be the judge. It is you who must decide. Are we so inviolate that we cannot be improved upon? Or are you willing to gamble on the intelligence of science to save us from the destruction science itself has bequeathed to us?

As you read this book, keep these questions in mind, for they lurk behind the excitement of every discovery: Right or wrong? Hope or disaster? Are we moving upward or marching to oblivion? I hope to convince you that up until now what psychopharmacology has done has been a net improvement. We have lifted mental illness out of the dark age of maltreatment, and we have helped millions of people get a toehold on life again. But as we head into the future, ethics loom large. We are close to tampering with the core of life. As Dr. Aryeh Routtenberg of Northwestern University said recently, "Some day we scientists are going to have to have a mind SALT talk."

This book is divided into four basic sections. The first deals with how we got where we are. It tells how we arrived at our present knowledge through a series of accidents that border on the freakish. The second part deals with how drugs really function—or at least how we presently *think* they function. It will explain simply and graphically what goes on in your head and what happens in your body when you take a tranquilizer.

The third section covers the "state of the art"—the most up-to-date theories concerning various disorders. We will discuss everything from depression to schizophrenia and describe the presently approved drug treatments.

Finally, we'll take a glimpse at the future—and I would ask that you read this part with particular detachment. We are only talking about possibilities, and I don't want to be accused of making wild-eyed predictions. About the only thing truly predictable in science is that nothing turns out the way anyone foresees. But the implications that confront us are both fascinating and critical, and I think it is very important that we all give some thought to them.

We are ready to begin a journey beyond Valium into a world landscaped by our psychology. It is a world where emotion is transformed into molecules, where mood and consciousness become physical mechanisms. I should warn you before we begin that some passages are technical. The human mind is a complicated chamber. Try as I may, I cannot reduce psychochemistry into an entertainment medium quite so accessible as a spy novel. Nevertheless, anyone can grasp it, and particularly those principles most relevant to our behavior. The reward for your labors will be a fuller understanding not only of drugs, but of the human condition.

2

A Trio of Accidents

In the late 1940s, so the story goes, a New York cab driver was heading south from Central Park. In his glove compartment was a bottle of pills his doctor had prescribed to combat hay fever. The period just following World War II, pharmaceutically speaking, was like a sideshow. We had all kinds of new remedies entering the marketplace, many of which had been used by the military. One of these new drugs was called antihistamine, which had been discovered in Europe some ten years earlier. This is what the cab driver had been using that day—an early forerunner of Contac and Dristan.

Antihistamines had one slight drawback. They were known to produce an occasional side effect. Patients were issued a standard warning not to use them while driving or operating machinery.

On that particular night a strange thing happened. The cab driver had only driven a mile or so when a police car pulled up and waved him to the curb. A patrolman got out carrying a book of summonses.

"You all right?" said the cop.

"Sure," said the hack. For the life of him he couldn't figure out what he had done wrong.

"Well, you just ran every red light for the last ten blocks," said the cop, "and either you're crazy as hell or you don't want to live too long."

Had the cab driver understood the significance of this event, he might have gone down in medical history, applauded as a second Isaac Newton, discovering the principle of gravity from a mishap with an apple tree. For science, it has been said, is the art of observation. Anybody can spill rubber and sulfur on a stove top, but if you miss the point that you have just invented tires, you won't get your name on a blimp over the Super Bowl.

All the poor cab driver got for his pains was a hefty fine to go with his hay fever. Presumably his doctor also missed the significance, as did thousands of other doctors who had heard similar stories.

What really happened was medically noteworthy: The cab driver had *not* fallen asleep at the wheel. He had seen and recorded every traffic light, but he had disobeyed them because *their significance seemed irrelevant to him!*

So the revolution began in the late 1940s with an unwanted side effect from a popular drug. The incident had been repeated many times. All that was needed was the right mind to recognize it.

"The development of drugs," a colleague once said, "is a classic example of medical ass-backwardness. Never once did we really know what we were developing. We just tried them, and if they worked, we considered ourselves geniuses." While that statement may be a little harsh, it nevertheless has validity. Drugs have been the products of trial and error; the major discoveries have been largely serendipitous.

But that might be said of *all* scientific breakthroughs. The major advances have never been orchestrated. Somebody notices something unusual and has the intelligence and curiosity to pursue the "why" of it. Dr. Seymour Kety, a leader in our specialty, has written with some acerbity about Nixon's War on Cancer. It was as if, said Kety, you could approach it militarily, with campaign maps, strategy and an arsenal full of test tubes. But if a US

President back in the nineteenth century had proclaimed, à la Nixon, a War on Mental Illness, we could not have advanced any faster than we were able to advance through random discovery. The reason for this is that we are chasing unknowns. Often we don't know the results we're looking for. We create a chemical, we try it on an animal, and only decades later might we spot the real value of it.

This was the way it was with antihistamines. We had created a drug that was supposed to cure sniffles. Only years later did it occur to anybody that the drug's unwanted "side effect" might actually be useful.

The earlier history of psychiatric drugs is long, tortuous and mostly frustrating. Although a number of sedatives and hypnotics were tried, none was successful nd many were dangerous. Freud himself expressed hope for cocaine. He not only prescribed it for patients but also tried it himself. The results of these experiments were predictably disastrous, and as a consequence drugs became distrusted by his followers.

The major share of credit for the drug revolution goes to an obscure French naval surgeon named Henri Laborit. He did not know much about psychiatry or Freud; but, like all great men, he had an obsession—he was determined to find a cure for surgical shock, the condition in which a patient on an operating table experiences a drop in blood pressure and his body stops functioning.

Laborit was convinced that this phenomenon could be prevented by improving the properties of anesthesia. He was looking for something that would keep the patient conscious but in a state of disinterest or "imperturbability."

That such a state existed had been known for centuries, probably since before the time of Homer. Helen of Troy was said to have served a drug that kept people awake but in a state of tranquility. The Greeks even had a word for this condition— *ataraxia*, meaning, literally, "to keep calm." If Laborit could find a drug that produced ataraxy, he was convinced it would be helpful in the surgical theater.

As he was pondering this problem from around the world came the reports of antihistamine. It was doing something strange—it

28

was making people drowsy. When it didn't make them drowsy, it was making them disinterested, putting an invisible wall between the user and the environment. Could it be that antihistamine was Laborit's solution? He was convinced that it was. The idea obsessed him. He began experimenting with various derivatives, but to no avail—there were too many possibilities.

About this time a large French pharmaceutical company became intrigued by Laborit and his magnificent obsession. What if he was right? Could you make a profit from it? Was it worth the investment that would be necessary to prove it? The Specia Company decided it was. They presented their staff with a mission impossible: to find Monsieur Laborit's magical elixir. If it didn't work in surgery, they would devise other uses for it.

To appreciate fully the results of this decision, you have to remember that postwar era. It was a time as psychiatrically different from the present as the Middle Ages was from the Age of Enlightenment. In 1948, in theaters around the world, audiences had been stunned by a movie called *The Snake Pit*. This movie depicted life in a mental institution with a despair that was vivid and, unfortunately, accurate. Life in those places was a waking nightmare. The disturbed were considered less than human. Since they were beyond the reach of any kind of healing, the only solution was complete isolation.

To show you the extent of how far we've come, in those days hospitals didn't even have psychiatric wards. It was unthinkable to allow a schizophrenic to share the same facilities as a heart patient or maternity case. When Dr. M. Ralph Kaufman built the first such mental ward at Mt. Sinai Hospital in 1948, it was an experiment bordering on revolution. Many a physician said no good would come of it.

Meanwhile in France, after months of experimenting, chemists synthesized a compound called 4560 RP. It seemed to meet many of Laborit's prerequisites, producing a state of ataraxy in various test animals. At a naval hospital called Val de Grâce, near the Mediterranean seaport of Toulon, France, a group of researchers decided to test 4560 RP to determine its effects on a mentally disturbed patient.

The patient's name was Jacques Lh. At twenty-four he was a

hopeless case. He had undergone so many insulin and electroshock treatments that he was a walking testimony to the failure of psychiatry. Then, at ten o'clock on a Saturday morning, January 19, 1952, Jacques Lh. made medical history. He was injected with 50 milligrams of 4560 RP.

Immediately Jacques began to calm down. He rested with his eyes shut, although he was fully conscious. The drug wore off after seven hours, and he was given another injection to obtain the same calming effect.

For ten days the battle between calm and agitation, the experimental compound and psychosis, dragged on. Jacques would rest, he would relax, he would eat and sleep, then suddenly the spasms and hallucinations would return. Finally the doctors began to notice a change. The periods of calm grew longer, more pervasive. On February 7 Jacques Lh. was pronounced "cured"— and a whole new era dawned on psychiatry.

A few years ago Dr. Jonathan Cole, a psychopharmacologist at Boston State Hospital, commented upon the irony that this greatest of discoveries has never been recognized by the Nobel Prize Committee. First, said Cole, the original discovery was made by a drug company rather than a university. This alone tended to tarnish the event, putting the spotlight on profits instead of research. Second, the drug was not conceived to help mental patients; it was conceived to prevent surgical shock, which it failed to do. Finally, Laborit, who had originally envisioned it, had neither the credentials nor the acumen to be elevated to hero status.

Nevertheless it was an astonishing discovery. Its social impact was almost immeasurable. Within three or four years it virtually emptied Europe's mental hospitals. And it created an explosion of research in psychochemistry.

I was a resident at Mt. Sinai at that time. I had graduated from medical school at the University of Nebraska. Like all young psychiatrists, I had been brought up on Freud, whose analytical principles were enshrined throughout the medical world. Particularly was this true in the United States. We were the haven for

30

Nazi Europe's oppressed. Disciples of Freud, fleeing internment and holocaust, found America the ideal recipient of their viewpoints.

And what brilliant people these Freudians were! They were thoughtful, incisive, they were imbued with humanism. If you had told them that their techniques were about to be replaced by a drug, you would have been assigned an internship in Outer Mongolia! Nevertheless, brilliant as they were, their analytical theories had one serious drawback: They might have helped a neurotic person gain self-awareness, but they never emptied a single hospital bed.

What was this compound, 4560 RP? They called it chlorpromazine—CPZ, for short. In America it assumed the brand name Thorazine. It is the granddaddy of all the antipsychotic drugs.

Ironically, as news of the CPZ discovery spread throughout Europe and reached America, it commingled with news of yet another "accident" that would have almost equally far-reaching effects. In this case it was a colleague of mine, a young psychiatrist named Nathan S. Kline, who would become the unwitting catalytic agent in a series of events that would have enormous significance.

One Sunday morning in 1953 Kline spotted an article in the *New York Times* that told how some psychiatrists in India had been experimenting with a plant root that had been rumored for centuries to contain "magical" properties. The name of this root was *Rauwolfia serpentina,* so labeled because of its snakelike appearance. It came from a shrub that grew in the mountains and was a popular item in the bazaars and marketplaces.

According to the article, *Rauwolfia serpentina* had been demonstrated to possess certain psychoactive properties. The benefits of the drug were not very clear, but there was evidence that it might help in the treatment of psychosis.

Kline was aware that there had been a similar report published years before, in 1931, but no one in the West had taken it seriously because we were still under the spell of the antidrug philosophy. What *was* taken seriously was that *Rauwolfia* might have medical value: There were encouraging reports that it controlled hypertension. Several American pharmaceutical companies were testing it as a drug to combat high blood pressure.

According to Kline's own published accounts, he became involved on the basis of a coincidence: He needed $500 for a new piece of lab equipment and was looking for a project to justify asking for it. He called a friend at Squibb Pharmaceuticals, which was one of the houses testing *Rauwolfia,* and a deal was struck in which Squibb would pay Kline to run additional tests of *Rauwolfia* on mental patients.

Kline described his tests in his book, *From Sad to Glad:*

> As a preliminary step four assistants and I took the drug for several weeks to test for safety. We tried both a preparation made from the plant root and a refined alkaloid extract called reserpine, which had been isolated in the interim by the Ciba Pharmaceutical Company. When we were reasonably sure that it would have no serious ill effects, we began a small trial with four patients. Two of them were schizophrenics and two were manic-depressives. The first results were not at all remarkable. There was clearly some sedative effect, but aside from becoming a little quieter, the patients showed no marked behavior change.
>
> At the next stage we enlarged the experiment to some 700 patients, taking in a broad range of cases from schizophrenics to psychoneurotics, and we started to increase the doses a bit at a time. Now some intriguing things began to happen. We found that in some cases the drug did affect behavior patterns.
>
> One of the patients studied in my private practice was a neophyte salesman who was so bound up by anxiety that he couldn't call on his customers. He hid out in movie theatres day after day in order to spare himself the humiliation of being turned down on an attempted sale. He knew that neglect of his job would catch up with him pretty fast, and that only increased his anxiety, but he couldn't force himself out of the self-defeating pattern.
>
> Under Rauwolfia medication he got the tension under manageable control and began to function. He wasn't

32

transformed suddenly into a successful salesman—indeed he was probably ill-suited for that calling—but at least he was able to get out on the street now and find out whether he could make sales or not.

At the time all this seemed very promising. Reserpine *(Rauwolfia)* enjoyed a brief popularity, but it was soon discovered to have a number of side effects, and it fell from grace as being inferior to Thorazine. But that didn't mean the story was over. The reserpine sensation created a change in the atmosphere. Particularly in America it put doctors on the alert that some new drugs might have mood-changing properties.

And that's when a most astonishing thing happened. Reserpine, as I've mentioned, was being used for high blood pressure. Suddenly it was noticed that many patients who were taking it were undergoing dramatic mood changes. In a word, they became "blue." They lost their appetite for life. They developed all the symptoms of clinical depression. They couldn't eat, they had disrupted sleep patterns, they felt encased in bell jars that deprived them of pleasure.

Try to imagine how shocking this was. As psychiatrists, our conditioning was strictly analytical. We viewed depression as hostility turned inward—something purely of the mind, not involving chemistry. Now we had an unexplained riddle. A plant root from India created all the same symptoms. Could it be that depression was chemically induced? Had those years of analysis been an exercise in futility?

The import was not lost on the scientific community. If depression was organic, so might be its antidote. The key to our emotions lay somewhere in our brain cells; it was a chemical entity; you could find it in a laboratory. Within the next ten years this hypothesis would appear valid. Studies would show that depression was inheritable, that a predisposition to it was locked into our genetic makeup and could be inherited like diabetes or baldness. Research would develop two different families of antidepressants—the MAO inhibitors and the tricyclics. And we would begin to probe deeper into the mysteries of electro-shock treatment, which to the Freudians of that era was a heretical therapy.

The third accident—and perhaps luckiest of all—actually ante-dates the discovery of chlorpromazine and reserpine, although it would not be accepted as scientifically valid until after those other drugs had changed our perspective.

The discovery of a new drug is like finding a needle in a haystack. The chances of success are less than one in ten thousand. Most chemists spend two-thirds of their lives in a laboratory and never come up with one marketable substance. The story I'm about to tell is about a man who defied those laws. He took one turn at bat and hit a home run. For this he earned not only the awe of his colleagues but more than a modicum of professional jealousy.

Among the most pernicious forms of mental illness is a category of disease called manic-depression. This is one of the so-called cyclical diseases, in that it involves recurring swings between euphoria and blackness. A number of famous people have been manic-depressives. It begins with a "high" and an increase of activity. Soon the victim is an unstoppable dynamo, unable even to sleep because of his or her energy and enthusiasm. This is followed by a crashing despondency, a gloom so thick that it is impossible to penetrate. It is a dangerous condition, highly self-destructive, and those who suffer from it rank right at the top of the potential-suicide chart.

One psychiatrist who became interested in this disease was an obscure Australian named John Cade. In the late forties Cade had evolved a hypothesis that manic-depression might be organic. He compared the disease to a condition like hyperthyroidism, in which an excessive natural substance imbalances the system. At the time this hypothesis seemed absurdly old-fashioned. In America he would have been scoffed at by the psychoanalytic establishment.

Following his presumption that the "poisons" might be natural, Cade reasoned that they must pass out of the body. Since the most likely escape route would be in the urine, this was where he began his research.

In a primitive laboratory of a small mental hospital, Cade took urine samples from a number of inmates. Some of these inmates were manic-depressives, but others were paranoid or schizophrenic. He injected the urine into a group of guinea pigs, which expressed their displeasure by keeling over dead. He noticed, however, that the manic-depressives' urine proved much more lethal at a lower dose level.

This finding only confirmed Cade's original hypothesis that there was a poison running loose in manic-depressives. He decided that the culprit might be uric acid, which over the years has caused so many problems for gout sufferers.

Taking the uric acid, which he feared might be too potent, Cade looked around for a solution in which to dilute it. On his shelf sat a bottle of lithium salts, a substance which was known to combine ideally with urates.

Lithium had been around since 1817. It was an alkali with a very undistinguished history. It had been tried unsuccessfully as a treatment for gout, then became a popular ingredient in folk medicines. During the 1940s it had been tried as a salt substitute, but it was so lethal that several patients died from it. In 1949—the same year as Cade's experiment—lithium was abandoned by the United States medical establishment.

Cade combined the urates with a lithium solution, filled a syringe and shot up some guinea pigs with it. He sat back to wait for the convulsions to start, just as they had in his previous experiment.

This time, however, there was a different outcome. The creatures just stared at him and looked mildly tranquil. Not only did the uric acid not kill them, they seemed actually relaxed and at peace with their environment!

Cade's has often been called a pure "dumb luck" discovery, but what happened next refutes that charge. There is nothing more seductive than one's own hypothesis, and it takes both courage and objectivity to have the willingness to scrap it. Cade's mind

35

seized quickly on the significant element: Never mind the hypothesis about urates; there was something in the lithium solution that manifested a remarkable behavior change.

Cade repeated the tests using a solution of lithium alone and found that the animals consistently became tranquil. Instead of struggling when he laid them on their backs, they seemed relatively content just to lie there and stare at him. Next he took some lithium and injected himself with it. Doctors have often done this as a preliminary toxicity test. In Cade's case he was lucky he survived, because an overdose of lithium can be highly toxic.

What Cade did next is truly extraordinary—beyond the bounds of all modern medicine—and illustrates why, in today's climate, a substance like lithium could not be so easily discovered. In order to perform a test in a hospital today, you must first go to a subcommittee on research. You must convince the committee members of the plausibility of your idea and that the test is worthy of consideration. From there the project goes to the hospital's research committee. The research committee mulls it over again. The members pass it along to the board of trustees, where it is given further debate and either passed or vetoed.

If a new drug is involved, the prospective researcher must submit the proposal to the Food and Drug Administration (FDA). Toxicity tests must be performed, and all the drug's effects must be weighed and analyzed. The whole process may take five or six years, and there is a good chance that the project will never come to pass at all. This is why many doctors complain that we have become cautious to the point of obstructing progress.

Cade never bothered to stand on such ceremony. He took his lithium and went to the hospital wards. He selected what he thought was a reasonable dosage, filled his syringe and injected ten patients with it.

As I've said, lithium is very toxic. Take too much and it will make you ill. On the other hand, if you don't take enough you will probably not get the results you are looking for. Patients on lithium must be constantly monitored. They receive periodic blood tests and adjustments of dosages. To take ten patients and to inject them arbitrarily was considered, even back then, a risky procedure.

Nevertheless, that is what John Cade did, and somehow, miraculously, he picked exactly the right dosage. As a group, the patients showed marked improvement—particularly those suffering from manic-depression. In the years ahead lithium became famous. It is one of the best-tailored drugs in our psychiatric arsenal. It flattens the mania in manic-depression and helps the patient keep her equilibrium.

So these were the breakthroughs that began to shake the world—chlorpromazine, reserpine and lithium carbonate. They revolutionized our attitude toward mental-health care and drove us full throttle into much-needed brain research. The revolution didn't just end there; it also spilled over into the so-called normal world. It reached into every doctor's office, every drugstore and ultimately into the public's medicine chests. For simultaneously with the development of these drugs came the development of other drugs with another kind of impact—drugs like Miltown, Librium, Valium and Dalmane, the so-called housewives' pills or minor tranquilizers. Although they are medically less significant, socially they have created a maelstrom. To unravel the mysteries surrounding these substances, it is appropriate to give them their own brief history.

3

The Birth of Valium

In May, 1957, Dr. Lowell Randall, director of pharmacology at Roche Laboratories in Nutley, New Jersey, was engaged in running tests on white mice, just as he had been doing routinely for years. Dr. Randall did not know it at the time, but today he was about to discover a gold mine. It would happen so subtly, so undramatically, that a lesser observer might have ignored it completely.

Ever since the CPZ discovery the drug business had been in a state of activity. There was fierce competition to find new mood changers, particularly those with tranquilizing properties. Roche, determined not to be left out, had alerted its chemists to this very objective. A profit-oriented subsidiary of Hoffmann-LaRoche in Switzerland, the company had an obligation to its stockholders to stay among the front-runners.

It was not only CPZ that motivated them. Down the road from Roche, in Cranberry, New Jersey, Wallace Laboratories, one of Roche's competitors, was sweeping the country with a product called Miltown. This was a brand-new type of tranquilizing agent, and its popularity with the public was both instant and unparalleled. It became a buzzword, a catch phrase, a sociological phenomenon—even Milton Berle used to make jokes on television about it. Of a chemical family called meprobamate (its identical twin carries the brand name Equanil), Miltown was the result of another scientific "accident," this one involving antibiotics. Penicillin, like antihistamine, was another of our many postwar "wonder drugs," but it soon became apparent that there were certain types of infectious bacteria that even megadoses of penicillin failed to neutralize. In 1945 Dr. Frank Berger, then a chemist with Wallace Laboratories, began investigating a number of substances in search of a chemical that would kill these bacteria. Among the many agents he and his co-workers tried was a marketed disinfectant called phenylglycol ether. They began tampering with this substance, rearranging its molecules, and they came up with a derivative, mephenesin carbamate.

They tested mephenesin on a group of white mice and found that although it didn't kill germs, it did make an excellent muscle relaxant. So what started out as an antibiotic was put on the market as a relaxant called Tolseram. Having noticed that this drug also seemed to allay anxiety, investigators changed Tolseram to intensify this effect. Some five years later, in 1955, we were introduced to the phenomenon of Miltown.

Miltown, unfortunately, had several drawbacks. It was very weak, requiring heavy dosage. A single pill contained up to 400 milligrams, meaning that on a per-milligram basis it was not efficacious. More disturbing, it made people drowsy. It was often used as a quasi-sleeping pill. For some people trying to function during the day, it created an unacceptable loginess.

Lowell Randall was aware of all this as he went about his work that day. His job was to supervise Roche's "basic screening tests," in which the effects of various chemicals were first observed in mammals. One of these tests was called the inclined screen test. It was a primitive little test, but brilliant in its simplicity. A wire mesh was leaned against a wall, and medicated white mice were encouraged to climb on it. The purpose of the test was to observe muscle-relaxing qualities. If the medication contained these properties, the rats couldn't climb. Their little legs would become loose and wobbly; they would lose their grip and slide down to the tabletop.

Up until then Dr. Randall had observed thousands of muscle relaxants, but in every case the results were the same. The mice would become weak, they would slide down the screen and within a very short time they would be either drowsy or unconscious. I mention this because it is important to understand the real method by which new drugs are "discovered." We usually credit the chemist—inaccurately—because of being the first to synthesize the compound. But chemists inevitably labor in darkness. They have no idea what effects their products will have. They live in a world of crystals and molecules, and the usefulness of their work must be judged by other people.

This was Dr. Randall's role. He tested the compounds the chemists provided him. These compounds arrived at his office by the hundreds and thousands, and most would get no further because they would be proved ineffective. But a substance arrived on this day called RO 5-0690. There was no reason to suspect that it was anything special. It was a compound that had been synthesized many years earlier by a chemist at Roche, Leo Sternbach.

A Polish immigrant graduated from the University of Krakow, Sternbach was something of a character around Roche. He was extremely dedicated and amazingly robust, and used to ski to work in winter when the roads were closed. In the twenty years he had been with Roche, he had never come up with a marketable compound. Like thousands of other chemists everywhere, he had spent a lifetime producing substances that were fallible.

In the 1930s, at the University of Krakow, Sternbach had become fascinated with "seven-member ring structures." These are a family of crystalline formations in which seven atoms are connected in a circle. He was not interested in the pharmacology of these structures; he was only interested in their theoretical aspects. He had made forty derivatives of these so-called heptoxdiazines, thirty-nine of which had proved perfectly useless.

Twenty years later, at his laboratory at Roche, Sternbach's

fortieth derivative sat gathering dust on a shelf. It had never been tried on any animal, and the odds were that it was just another failure. Then, while cleaning up one day, one of Sternbach's assistants noticed the bottle. Realizing that the derivative had never been tested, they sent it over to Randall's office and forgot all about it.

To Randall, RO 5-0690 was just another chemical that probably wouldn't work. Or if it did work, it would work in all the wrong ways, and he would be left trying to figure out what you could use it for. Trial and error, trial and error. It is a difficult, painstaking, rather boring procedure. A researcher lives for something new, something that doesn't fit the predictable pattern.

Randall took a group of mice, injected them with the compound and set them on the screen to see how they would behave. Would they be able to climb? Would they fall off in a coma? Or would they just behave as if nothing had happened? It soon became apparent that whatever this agent was, it did have some sort of relaxant effect. This alone seemed to make it unique, since previous heptoxdiazines had been proven to be inert. The mice began to lose their grip. Their legs weakened and they slid down the screen. They were as relaxed as if they had been given a barbiturate—or, for that matter, a good strong dose of Miltown.

But science is based upon the observation of differences. The replication of sameness means you have succeeded at nothing. It is only the unique, the unexpected, that makes one's heart pulse with the thrill of discovery. And that's the sensation Lowell Randall must have felt. Something was different—the chain of sameness had been broken. For instead of falling asleep, these mice were wide awake. Even in their weakness they had lost little of their alertness.

Word spread quickly throughout the laboratories at Roche, which are almost always alive with the rumor of some new "miracle." Somebody has just discovered a cure for cancer, or there's some amazing new elixir that seems to eliminate labor pains. Usually, of course, these hopes are soon dashed. The observation can't be substantiated, or there are problems in the toxicity tests. Every scientist is a would-be Pasteur, just as every

41

actor is a would-be Marlon Brando. But there was something different about Sternbach's compound—and that, in Randall's eyes, was the significant factor. It would need further testing, further analysis, but it had all the earmarks of a pharmacological breakthrough.

What was this compound? In physical terms it was a colorless powder, highly soluble in water. It seemed to require protection from light, and it was very unstable when placed in solution. Its generic name was *chlordiazepoxide*. It belonged to a family called *benzodiazepines*. Three years later it would be marketed as a pill, and the public would come to know it by its brand name, Librium.

That Librium was potentially superior to Miltown was evident to the executives at Roche from the outset. In the first place, it was shown to be extraordinarily nontoxic, and that would make it attractive for marketing. Dr. Albert Zobel, retired director of communications at Roche and a member of Librium's initial study team, recalls that "we could give an animal almost any amount of Librium and all it would do is sleep for a few hours." The reason for this was that, unlike barbiturates, Librium did not depress the respiratory system. This meant that doctors could prescribe it with impunity, setting aside their concerns about suicides and overdoses.

Librium's first outside test came at the San Diego Zoo. One of the veterinarians there had made an appeal to Roche. The zoo had just acquired a new Siberian tiger that was acting vicious and resentful of captivity. This is a perpetual problem for zoos: Many new animals are both rare and expensive, and when they are first captured and placed in cages, they can go wild to the point of self-destruction. Traditional sedatives were not working well; the animals would grow drowsy and refuse to eat. What was needed was a tranquilizer that would calm the beast yet keep it conscious and alert so people could look at it.

Roche sent out a supply of Librium. Within days the veterinarian was calling excitedly. Not only had Librium calmed the tiger down, the beast was so good-natured she would let you play with her!

Perhaps here I should insert an observation about the deceptive nature of animal testing. Animals and humans are not only built differently, we also don't have the same behavior patterns. I have noticed that people sometimes get confused when they read an account about a new medical "breakthrough," then are told further down that the drug cannot be marketed yet because the results have only been observed in animal studies.

Let me relate a case out of my own file of memories. Several years ago there was a drug we'll call X, which, when administered to a group of animals, seemed to have all the earmarks of an antidepressant. Then came time to test it on humans. We took two volunteers who were deeply depressed. We gave them each an injection of X and sat back to see what results it would have on them.

Well, what happened was truly unexpected. They didn't become cheerful, they became uncontrollably manic! They began to chatter in a nonsensical fashion and to scribble all over the walls of their hospital rooms. As the doctor in charge, I was alarmed, then horrified. We had turned two depressed patients into hallucinating psychotics. I am happy to report that as a result of such experiments, the drug in question never got to the marketplace.

And so it might have been with Librium. It worked beautifully on tigers and zebras and dingos, but everyone knew that if the drug was to succeed it would have to take that step out of the veterinary sciences.

Librium's acid test came in 1960, when samples of it were sent to a clinic in Texas. The psychiatrists there were asked to try it on patients and report its effect as an antianxiety agent. Clinicians are slow. They are given hundreds of drugs and asked to evaluate them. Usually their replies are somewhat less than inspiring, with a lot of "ifs" and "perhapses" and other qualifications. But in this case the response was swift and dramatic. A letter was forwarded to the president of Roche. Whatever this new drug is, the letter said in effect, you'd better make more of it, because its success is astonishing!

Well, this was undoubtedly good news to Roche. A drug like this could involve a very high profit margin. But it would take one

43

more piece of evidence to convince the marketing department that this was a drug worth pulling out all the stops for.

As it happened, one of the executives at Roche (who for obvious reasons will remain anonymous) was confronting one of life's seamier problems—a critical case of mother-in-law-itis. The woman was impossible. She was irritable and cranky, and she made everyone she encountered a nervous wreck. She was infamous throughout the top echelons of Roche. People would do anything to avoid being at dinner parties with her.

The executive obtained some Librium from the laboratory. He confronted the virago with an innocuous suggestion: perhaps she would like to try some of these new pills, which seemed to be beneficial for "sensitive" temperaments. The woman agreed. She began to take Librium. The change in her behavior was instant and extraordinary. In one fell swoop the executive saved his home life and put the final zing into Roche's promotional efforts.

News of Librium spread swiftly throughout the medical community. Requests poured in from all over the world. Every researcher wanted to run evaluations of it, every MD wanted to allay his patients' complaints with it. Thus the seeds of its abuse, perhaps, were sown from the outset. Later critics would accuse Roche of hyped promotion, but Roche would counter, with some justification, that it was word of mouth by doctors that was responsible for the Librium boom.

Meanwhile Sternbach, undaunted by all this controversy, reported for work every day at the laboratory. Having given the world one new antianxiety agent, he was busily determined to give it yet a better one.

For those of you who have taken basic chemistry, Dr. Sternbach's world might not seem so mysterious; it is a world governed by the invisible and unknowable; we can only see the outward effects of it. Unlike biology, where with the aid of a microscope even the smallest cells become palpable entities, the structure of chemicals is so infinitesimal that the configurations remain theoretical. You can only know them by the results of tests. You apply certain agents that will redefine the structure. Through the visible reactions, you can then form hypotheses as to the probable appearance of the molecules you are dealing with.

44

So the ring structure that so fascinated Sternbach was an abstraction, a theory, a visionary's concept. Ring structures had first been postulated in 1865 by a chemist named Friedrich Kekule, to whom they had literally appeared one night in a dream. He had pictured serpents lying in a circle, all holding on to one another's tails. He had awakened realizing that this was how atoms might lock. Subsequent tests have verified this hypothesis.

During the months ahead Sternbach and his co-workers produced thousands of seven-member ring structures. Many of them proved to be clinically effective, but none was superior to the original Librium. Then one day they found the exception. Its generic name was *diazepam*. In 1963 it was marketed as Valium, and for millions it would become either a curse or a savior.

Valium—the name is derived from Latin and means literally "to be strong and well"—is the most frequently prescribed drug in medical history, with prescriptions in the United States totaling almost 39 million. When it hit the market, Hoffmann-LaRoche's stock quadrupled, soaring from about 50,000 gold francs to almost 200,000. Within the next few years it captured half the tranquilizer market, and Valium became synonymous with all anxiolytics. It is a remarkable drug in that it does more than relieve anxiety. Surgeons use it as a muscle relaxant. It is also used to treat certain forms of epilepsy and, in undeveloped countries, as a therapy for tetanus.

Intrinsically Valium is no better than Librium—they both achieve fairly similar effects—but Valium is the more potent of the two and, as a muscle relaxant, has greater versatility. Primarily the choice is one of personal preference, depending on one's individual chemistry. But since Valium has become the more popular drug, it has also become the target of broadest criticism.

So much debate has been stirred around these pills that the subject cannot be addressed simplistically. A lot depends on personal prejudices and the values with which we were raised as children. I happen to be rather conservative on the subject. I think most cases do not call for tranquilizers. The use of tranquilizers tends to lead to a desire for instant gratification, and I believe this can be psychologically destructive. Life is built around both pleasure and pain. They are the poles of our existence; they

45

are what drive and motivate us. When you seek pleasure without being willing to endure its opposite, you are frustrating one of nature's most basic mechanisms. The taking of a tranquilizer is the denial of pain. It is an attempt to grab the cheese without running the maze. That doesn't work with mice, and it won't work with us, either. We need hardship and striving to develop inner strength.

Surveys sponsored by pharmaceutical houses have turned up a widespread "Calvinism" toward tranquilizers. That is, there are many people who think that the use of Valium is immoral and provides false security while weakening will power. While I wish that some of the people who have these prejudices would be willing to extend them to other drugs, like alcohol, I generally applaud this as a healthy response, and I would not for one moment wish to imply that it is foolish. But I do not believe that moral rectitude is a legitimate excuse for endangering one's life. When tension and anxiety begin seriously to impair us, the use of mood changers may be justified on a short-term basis.

Admittedly, this is somewhat arbitrary. Who is to say what is a "serious impairment"? Is it a month of depression? A rocky marriage? Or must we wait until a person makes a couple of suicide attempts? I don't have the answer to this. Each individual has her or his own psychic threshold. What is annoying to one may be devastating to another, and I lack the divinity to affix a firm boundary line.

Personal attitudes and cultural conditioning are fairly well reflected in the people who use tranquilizers. Some 65 percent are women—just as about 65 percent of most doctors' patients are female. This has led to a paranoid suspicion that perhaps the use of tranquilizers is a sexist plot; that perhaps doctors, mostly being men, are seeking psychic revenge, and find chemical sedation a convenient way of doing this. While I'll admit that recent changes in our society have created male-female strains that didn't used to be there, I see no evidence of a plot among doctors to keep women patients in chemical straitjackets. Rather, if there is a problem, I think it may be on the patients' side. Too many women look at pills as therapy. The highest incidence of prescriptive-drug abuse is among female patients who are forty and over.

A majority of these pills are not prescribed by psychiatrists. They are prescribed by general practitioners and specialists. A recent survey in a major New York hospital revealed that only 10 percent of minor tranquilizers were being prescribed by psychiatrists. This would seem to mean that there is a large network of professionals who may be prescribing pills for vaguely psychiatric reasons. If there is a patient who can't sleep or who has a nebulous nervous complaint, the doctor is tempted to scribble out a Valium prescription. This is not only human, it is probably inevitable. In doctors, presumably, there is a desire to help people. If you have a drug as tested as Valium, it seems both humane and practical to make patients feel better with it.

On the other hand, this is what leads to abuse. Doctors may prescribe the drug a little too willingly. They may see it as a "shortcut" to relieve the patient's misery, without inquiring properly into the underlying causes. Use of tranquilizers can often mask deep psychological problems, which is another reason Freudians have traditionally been wary of them: In analysis anxiety is considered useful; the well-relaxed patient can present too many obstacles. Valium is at best a Band-Aid treatment and as such has severe limitations. You can't keep applying bandages to a wound that has become festering and gangrenous beneath the skin.

Happily this practice is already on the decline; in the past five or six years there has been a drop-off in the number of Valium prescriptions. In fact, all minor tranquilizers are less prescribed now, and there has been an overall tightening in the number of refills allowed. But this doesn't mean the practice won't continue—it will almost have to continue because of the demands of our society. As long as there are so many anxiety-ridden people out there, nonpsychiatric professionals will be called upon as auxiliary forces.

At a number of hospitals there has been such concern that the question has been raised as to whether we should limit tranquilizer prescriptions. It has been asked in staff meetings whether we should place heavier restrictions on tranquilizer prescriptions by other than psychiatrists. In the majority of cases this has been rejected. Tranquilizers have too many legitimate uses. They play a positive role in many situations, and to place arbitrary controls on them does not seem constructive. Medicine's official position— with which I agree—is that we need better education for both doctors *and* consumers. Tranquilizers, like automobiles, are here to stay, and the only way to live with them is to develop respect for them.

Be that as it may, how dangerous is Valium?* How worried should we be about its effects on our bodies? Is it destroying our society? Can it rob us of our will? Is it inherently harmful for having been produced in a laboratory? These are not easy questions to answer. None of them deserves a simple yes or no answer. And, given the general level of skepticism today, even if I answered them simply, no one would believe me. So let's address them one at a time, looking at the facts as objectively as possible. Keep in mind that we are talking about our *present* knowledge, not projected problems that have yet to be unearthed.

First: Can Valium kill you? This is an important question, because whatever merits a drug might have, if there's a danger of taking it and dropping dead, its overall attractiveness is greatly diminished. The question has added piquancy today in view of cases like that of Karen Ann Quinlan, for whom tranquilizers mixed with a large quantity of alcohol caused a grotesque suspension between life and oblivion.

The National Institute of Drug Abuse has a subsidiary arm, the Drug Abuse Warning Network (DAWN), which in recent years has issued annual reports that have implicated Valium in a number of fatalities. Most of these fatalities are "Valium associated"—that is, Valium was used along with something else. But in some forty to fifty cases a year, Valium has been listed as the only cause of death.

Institutions like DAWN perform a valuable service. They

---

*"Valium" in the discussion that follows is interchangeable with all minor tranquilizers, including: Librium, Dalmane, Miltown, Equanil, Ativan, Vistaril, Atarax, Serax and others. The chemical properties are not all alike, but their effects are such that similar precautions should be exercised in the use of all of them.

increase our awareness of drug abuse. Drugs are seducers; they are like loaded pistols, and if you don't respect them you are bound to be hurt by them. But one of the requisites of being a scientist is learning to spot the deceptiveness of statistics. Statistics can lie, even if their compilers don't mean them to, and journalists can pervert them for the sake of a scare story.

One of the problems with the DAWN reports is that they don't call attention to *all* the statistics. One, for example, that is frequently obscured is the ratio between prescriptions and fatalities. Take 1977, for example. The report for that year is not the latest available, but it received wide circulation through various media, and it's as good a year as any to focus upon. In 1977, says DAWN, fifty fatalities resulted from Valium alone. There were another nine hundred in which Valium was implicated, having been found in the bodies along with other substances. On the face of it this is a disturbing statistic. Nine hundred and fifty deaths has a headline ring to it. It's as if every year the medical profession were implicitly condoning the self-destruction at Jonestown.

But an examination of the complete statistics reveals that there were more than 57 million Valium prescriptions written that year. That's almost twice as many as for the number-two drug, Darvon, which was involved in 1,420 fatalities. Moreover, Darvon was the only drug in use in 320 cases. Its death-to-prescription ratio is about 1 in 100,000. Valium's, on the other hand, is about 1 in 1,000,000—making it ten times as safe using DAWN's own statistical base.

But how were these statistics gathered? Who were these victims, and who did the analyzing? If you don't know how the numbers were compiled, you don't have any basis upon which to judge them.

DAWN gets its statistics from medical examiners' offices, which is logical because that's where autopsies are performed. Reports are filed on a voluntary basis, and there is a considerable disparity in both their quality and completeness. Some cities have very up-to-date laboratories; others get by on a minimum of equipment. When the reports come to DAWN, they are all treated equally. There is little or no attempt to verify their accuracy.

49

Since these reports come from coroners' offices, one of the chief causes of death is apparent suicide. This means we are dealing with emotionally wounded people, and that helps explain why there are so many tranquilizers involved. It is not unusual, when dealing with suicides, to find that many of them have been on medication. When you have a drug as popular as Valium, what could be less surprising than to find many appearances of it? But this doesn't mean that Valium killed these people. It only means that it was found in their bodies. The coroner might also have found arsenic and a gunshot wound, but the death will be listed as "Valium associated."

There are other problems with gathering statistics this way. Many of the reports don't quantify dosage. Are we talking about one tablet or six, or a handful of them? What amount constitutes a lethal overdose? Valium, you see, has some unusual properties, one of them being an extremely long "half-life." It will remain in the body for many days, long after other substances are eliminated. It is also unusually easy to detect, because traces can be measured to the billionth of a milligram. Few other substances are so readily traceable, and certainly not after they have had time to be metabolized.

A far more reliable study than DAWN's was one conducted by Dr. Bryan S. Finkle, a toxicologist with the University of Utah who decided to conduct his own nationwide survey. Between August and November, 1976, Finkle and his associates visited twenty-seven medical examiners' offices throughout the United States and Canada, in communities representing 79.2 million people. In the three years covered by the parameters of their study, they came up with 1,500 Valium-related deaths. Some of these cases were drownings and automobile accidents, in which Valium was only mentioned as being possibly contributory.

The most frequent manner of death was suicide. In these cases, there were usually other drugs present—sometimes a barbiturate, sometimes alcohol—often consumed in a prodigious quantity. Of the fifty-one cases involving alcohol and Valium, for example, 75 percent showed an enormous alcohol consumption. Only two

50

deaths showed an unusually high Valium concentration where the alcohol level was less than 0.10 percent.

The bottom line of Finkle's report is that there were only two cases in which Valium alone was suspect. Even in those two cases the evidence wasn't conclusive, but no other substance was found that could have caused death. Two cases in all the United States and Canada. Two cases out of millions of prescriptions. That is a remarkable statistic indeed, and it has been corroborated by similar studies in other countries.

So now we can see how Valium became so popular: It is one of the few prescribed medicines that is virtually suicide proof. That is a major consideration for any doctor dispensing pills for a mental or emotional problem. This is why barbiturates fell into disfavor— it was too easy for patients to do themselves in with them. While doctors try to tell themselves that they are not to blame for this, it is a heavy responsibility for any physician to live with.

As relatively safe as Valium is, however, this doesn't mean it can be used with abandon. On the contrary, it is a very potent drug, figuring in more than fifty thousand emergency-room cases annually. The problem with Valium is that it becomes an additive to other drugs—it may even "potentiate" or multiply the effects of them. When taken with alcohol or some other depressant, Valium seems to encourage the other drugs' sedative effects.

Why this is we're really not sure. We do know that depressants work on the central nervous system and that while Valium alone has little effect on this system, it encourages other drugs to become even more devastating. Your central nervous system controls your breathing. This is a partially autonomic activity. When you combine Valium with another depressant, you can slip into unconsciousness and your lungs may stop functioning.

Maybe it's best to think of Valium this way: It is like a docile dog which, when left on its own, causes very few problems that can't be cured and may at times even be considered helpful toward its master. But let that same dog run free with other dogs and it can quickly turn into a vicious accomplice. In this case the other dogs are alcohol and barbiturates, which, in Valium's company, become extremely dangerous.

51

Aside from fatality, doesn't Valium cause other problems? Doesn't it lead to addiction and dependency? Aren't I better off trying to cope by myself rather than hobbling through life using chemicals as a crutch?

Few experts in this field would disagree with that. You might say Valium is a victim of its own success. It has been overheralded and overprescribed, and there have been a number of patients who have persisted in abusing it. Dr. Sidney Cohen of the University of California in Los Angeles puts the problem in proper perspective, I think, when he writes that "mild tension or appropriate situational anxiety is not an indication for any psycho-chemical." I think some doctors in the past have failed to grasp this. Patients should learn how to cope by themselves. There are many ways of alleviating anxiety without running to the medicine cabinet in search of a "feel-good" pill.

One of the problems many doctors have had is that they prescribe a tranquilizer, then lose touch with the patient. The patient goes on getting refill after refill without anyone present to warn of impending catastrophe. In Valium's case the problem has been worse, because some pharmacists have been lulled into relaxing their standards. Knowing that the drug is so nontoxic, they have sometimes winked at requests for refills instead of challenging them.

In an attempt to combat this, in 1975 the government upgraded Valium to a "Schedule IV" drug. This means that renewals cannot exceed five within the six months following the first prescription. Some say that the drug should be upgraded still further. I'm inclined to agree with this position. I am very leery of authorizing refills by telephone, and I will usually insist that the patient come in for a visit first.

With regard to Valium's addictiveness and dependency problems, let's first define what we mean by those terms. They are not synonymous, and it is important not to get them confused. *Addiction* is a physical state in which the body has adjusted to a chemical additive. When you withhold the additive, you suffer withdrawal symptoms—muscle spasms, dry mouth, convulsions, whatever. *Dependency*, on the other hand, is psychological. It is the profoundly perceived need to continue a habit. This happens when the pleasure we derive becomes so indispensable that to deny ourselves is emotionally uncomfortable.

Cigarette smoking creates both addiction and dependency. If you give up the habit you will suffer mild withdrawal symptoms. Your heart rate will change, your mouth will salivate, you may feel a number of sensations that are very real and palpable. But you will also hunger psychologically. You will feel deprived of an activity that has "enhanced" your life. You may have to make certain social and work adjustments to bring yourself in line with the nonsmoking image of yourself.

Valium has been proven to create both addiction and dependency. An estimated 15 percent of users may have experienced one or the other of these problems. In my practice I have seen a number of Valium addicts. They have come to me after years of abuse. They are taking 20 to 40 or more milligrams a day, and their bodies literally can't get along without the stuff. When you take them off it, you see visible symptoms—twitching hands and muscle spasms. This may last a couple of weeks, followed by a gradual easing of tension. It takes about a month to get a person off Valium, and it can be a very difficult and unpleasant experience. The usual way is to wean the patient gradually, reducing the dosage a few milligrams at a time.

Valium, like all tranquilizers, can also cause dependency. Some users may feel insecure if they don't have their pills with them. They may be in such fear of whatever *bête noire* is chasing them that they will down pill after pill in an attempt to vanquish it. In this regard Valium is not unlike alcohol. In some instances liquor is not physiologically addictive, but it can create a dependency so subtle and profound that the drinker will refuse to face what is happening. Dependency is in some ways worse than addiction, in that it is easier for the victim to make excuses for it. "I don't really *need* it," the person may argue, "but I enjoy it, and therefore I can continue doing it."

I can foresee a day when we may solve our addiction problems, because that's a physiological process and subject to alteration. What is created by chemistry can presumably be uncreated by it, and research is already being done in this area. But dependency is far more subtle and pernicious. It can only be eliminated through behavior modification. The best defense is a preventive posture, which means not to let yourself be enslaved in the first place.

Hand in hand with addiction and dependency is another problem that we call *drug tolerance*. This is when increasing amounts of a drug deliver less and less of the result you are seeking. We don't really know what causes tolerance, although it could be related to a change in cell structure, but we do know that it occurs with a wide range of drugs, and Valium and Librium are no exceptions. This means that when you first take one of these tranquilizers, the initial effects may seem quite miraculous, but as you continue using it day after day, you may need more and more just to maintain equilibrium.

Dr. Arthur K. Shapiro, formerly of the Payne Whitney Psychiatric Clinic but now on staff at Mt. Sinai Hospital, has just completed a study on Valium that underscores the problem of tolerance. He took 224 anxious outpatients and assigned some to Valium, some to placebo. He then constructed a complex protocol that would identify factors not related to Valium effect.

The results of this study were most enlightening. He found that *Valium is not superior to placebo after the first week of treatment!* From that point on any effects you feel are the same effects that you would get from a sugar pill!

Is it true that Valium is being sold as a "street drug"?

Yes, and for quite large sums, I'm told. This is not an area in which I am an authority, but it has helped worsen the drug's reputation.

In the street culture Valium is what is known as a downer. Drug users are not very sophisticated about chemistry. They group Valium and barbiturates together as downers, while amphetamines and others are referred to as uppers. Scientifically speaking, this is meaningless nomenclature. It doesn't even reflect the drugs' true activities, but for the illicit purposes these people have in mind, I suppose it's accurate enough and not worth arguing over.

One of the purposes for which street people use Valium is to counteract the effects of a "bummer." People who use amphetamines—otherwise known as speed freaks—will keep Valium around to ease the horrors of "crashing." Valium has also shown up among methadone users, creating considerable interference in many of our treatment centers. Some of the doctors who have been most critical of Valium are those who have seen its effects in drug clinics.

Valium has also been used to treat alcoholism. The dried-out alcoholic may become tense and agitated. Valium is used to relax these people and sometimes to quell their soured combativeness.

Don't we Americans take too many tranquilizers?

Yes, we do, and I think that is cause for concern. We are ordering 38.5 million Valium prescriptions a year and more than 60 million of all minor tranquilizers. On the other hand, as I have said, this is down considerably from 1974, the peak year for tranquilizers, when Valium prescriptions reached more than 60 million and total minor-tranquilizer prescriptions were over 100 million.

But tranquilizers are not just an American problem. That is another area where we tend to delude ourselves. We think that anything trendy belongs to us, and that when the world goes to hell they'll find the United States waiting for them. The National Institute of Drug Abuse, curious about world attitudes toward tranquilizers, conducted a study among nine European countries, with results that many Americans might find surprising. Far from being a leader in tranquilizer use, America ranks fairly close to the middle, ahead of Spain but behind France and Belgium, neither a leader nor a prodigal, on the whole fairly conservative. Perhaps this is because of our Puritan background. I mentioned earlier our Calvinistic attitudes. Most Americans are not quite as trusting as we think, and I see little evidence that we will all become drug addicts.

Nevertheless, I must emphasize the dangers of these drugs and the amount of respect a patient should show toward them. I would urge every reader to follow this checklist of contraindications religiously:

Don't take tranquilizers if you are driving a car. While Valium is not as bad as its predecessors, it can make some people very drowsy, and it is wise to stay away from all dangerous machinery.

Don't take alcohol if you are taking Valium or any other sedative-type drug. You may be surprised what two martinis can do when mixed with two 5-milligram Valium tablets.

Never mix drugs without consulting a doctor—and always tell the doctor what drugs you are taking. One plus one is not always two. In the case of drugs it can be ten, and lethal.

Don't take Valium if you are pregnant. In fact, this is a good rule to extend to all drugs. Valium readily crosses the placental barrier, with effects on the fetus that we have not fully explored yet.

Don't take Valium if you are over 65, unless you are following a doctor's orders. Among the elderly Valium can have a "paradoxical reaction" and can make some people highly and perhaps dangerously agitated.

Don't exceed the daily recommended dosage. Usually this is from 2 to 20 milligrams. The average dose is about 15 milligrams. If you exceed these numbers you may land in trouble.

Do not use Valium for more than one or two weeks. It should only be used for short-term crises. And don't go back on it until you have talked to a doctor and have determined that it is safe to do so.

In the next chapter we're going to show how drugs affect the human brain. In the meantime I would like to leave you with this thought which appeared several years ago in the *New York Times Magazine.* Author Gilbert Cant, analyzing our fears about Valium, noted that the drug is "generating as much anxiety as it was meant to allay." If Valium has become something we rely on in our hedonistic culture, he wrote,

. . . its use is a symptom rather than a cause of this condition. Properly used by the medical profession, Valium has only medicinal properties. A drug has no moral or immoral qualities. These are the monopoly of the user or abuser.

4

The Psychic Tennis Game

Have you ever found yourself suffering from an emotion when your conscious mind seems totally unaware of it? That is, you feel angry, depressed, anxious or tense, yet your response will be to deny that anything is troubling you? Of course you have; it's common to all of us. Television commercials blame it on caffeine. In real life the problem may be much more complex, involving some very interesting psychiatric hypotheses.

Let's take a typical domestic situation. You and your spouse are having dinner, the children are playing in another room and as far as you know, you are behaving naturally. Suddenly your spouse says, "Why are you upset?"

You say, "Upset? Who's upset? I'm not upset."

Your spouse says, "Yes, you are. Your cheeks are flushed, and you're attacking your food as if it were some sort of enemy."

What do you suppose is behind that reaction? How could you be angry and not even know it? Why should your hands and cheeks and heart rate be responding to something of which you are consciously unaware?

Ever since the earliest days of science, one question has always troubled philosophers: Where do we get these feelings called emotions? Where do they originate and why do they trouble us so? Aristotle thought he had the answer. Emotions, he hypothesized, arise from the heart. Others blamed the circulatory system, or "humors" that emanated from the liver or bile duct.

It wasn't until 1937 that an obscure scientist named James Papez set forth the concept that our emotions, our *feelings*, originate from a circuit buried deep within the brain. This circuit, he theorized, is very complex. It is not a solitary structure. Rather it involves a series of structures that act as a conduit between consciousness and the rest of the body.

If you were to ask a person what triggered his emotions, he would probably respond that they originated in the mind. He would say that the trembling or heat change in his body was a response to an idea his mind had formulated. There is a contradictory theory, however, that holds that the body may "know" first, and that the mind follows later. Put another way: you are not running because you are afraid; rather you are afraid because you have learned that you are running.

This theory, which is called the James-Lange hypothesis, has never been substantiated by empirical evidence, but it gains a certain plausibility when viewed in context with Papez and his "emotional circuit." The theory implies a two-way process: input from the body is passed up to the consciousness, while input from the consciousness is passed down to the lower organs, and it's anybody's guess as to which was the initiator. These impulses pass through the Papez circuit, also called the *limbic system*. Its responses can activate many biochemical processes.

Marcel Proust, in *Remembrance of Things Past*, was aroused by the smell of warm tea and madeleines. The odors transported him into a maelstrom of emotions, which he subsequently translated into conscious memories. Proust didn't know it, but his limbic system did that. In animals, this system is reliant on smell. It is the seat of the so-called fight-or-flight response, and it plays a critical role in survival and sex arousal.

The human limbic system is similar to that of animals, only we have evolved to the point that we can think further than our noses. We know how to translate ideas and abstractions, and we depend more on our eyesight than on our olfactory system. Nevertheless, we do have a limbic system, and in our brain it also controls emotions and sex. As such it has drawn a great deal of research— particularly its role in the so-called mood disorders.

Once we discovered this sytem's existence and learned how it might color our various nerve impulses, we got our first inkling of how abstract thought processes might be intimately entwined with physical anatomy. The limbic system influences both feelings and actions. Control of emotions is achieved through the involuntary nervous system; actions are under the control of the voluntary nervous system which may or may not possess the power to inhibit them. This gives a new dimension to the precepts of Freud: We now have a location in which to place the unconscious, making it a network of nerve tracts that can both act and respond without any cognition.

To some people this is an unsettling idea. It was bad enough when Freud said that we were programmed by our experiences. At least he left us some psychological abstractions that we could choose to translate in terms of the spirit. The new hypothesis doesn't even leave us that. It says that our unconscious is a matrix of nerve cells. It pushes us further toward a mechanistic outlook in which we may view ourselves as complex machines.

To pick up the illustration from the start of this chapter, as you talk to your spouse, your body gets "angry." Something has triggered a *physiological* response, and it is only later that you become consciously aware of it. Perhaps a parallel has already occurred to you: This is not unlike what we discovered with reserpine. A chemical or substance that affects the body can subsequently trigger a change in one's psychic state.

Armed with the aforementioned trio of drug discoveries and the Papezian hypothesis about the limbic system, scientists began to scrutinize brain cells for telltale links between chemistry and thought processes. It did not take long for an answer to appear. We discovered something called *neurotransmitters*. The discovery of these substances has revolutionized psychiatry and launched a twenty-year probe into the brain's smallest particles.

To understand what neurotransmitters are and the role they may play in both mood and cognition, it is necessary to know how a nerve cell works and the function it has within a neuronal network. Do you remember the old Frankenstein movies? The scientist always had a beaker with a human brain in it. It was suggested that the brain was kept alive by chemicals and could be activated by electricity that came down through a lightning rod. Well, that was partially correct. The brain does contain chemicals, and electrical currents do make it operate; only it cannot survive in a tank full of fizz water, and we do not have to be hooked up to lightning rods or wall outlets.

The brain contains many, many billions of nerve cells. Estimates run as high as fifty billion or more. Each of these cells is connected with other cells via many hundreds of wispy filaments. According to the National Academy of Sciences, the complexity of this one organ is beyond anything imaginable. "A single human brain," they write, "has a greater number of possible connections among its nerve cells than the total number of atomic particles in the universe."

Each of these nerve cells carries a charge of electricity, which is simply the movement of very small particles. This movement is chemical, as it is in a battery, created by two different substances with differing charge values. The chemicals in our nerve cells are sodium and potassium. Sodium is on the outside, potassium is on the inside. They are separated by a thin, semi-permeable membrane, which is molecularly transformed as the chemicals pass through it.

If you compared a nerve cell to a soccer field, the cell would look like a team trying to set up a goal. Much of the movement is from side to side, but the resulting momentum is inexorably forward. It looks like *Figure 1*, page 62.

This activity can be triggered by a number of causes. Some of these, we now know, are psychological. This is part of the new mechanistic view, and, as I said before, the implications are unsettling.

61

FIGURE 1
How Electricity Travels Through a Nerve Cell

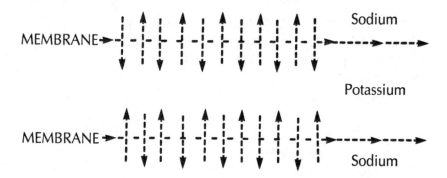

If our nerve cells can be compared to soccer fields, what happens between those cells is more like tennis—only the volleys are so quick and flawless that it would take a lifetime to sort out the many interplays. The "balls" are those molecular substances called *neurotransmitters*. They are the detonators that trigger our nerve cells to fire. They fly back and forth between one cell and another, sailing over a channel which is called a *synapse*.

We think there may be as many as two hundred different transmitter types, but so far we have identified fewer than two dozen. Each transmitter has its own generic shape and is tailored to fit cells found in particular kinds of nerve tracts. The transmitters are manufactured by various enzymes. Similarly, there are other enzymes that metabolize, or destroy, them. As in everything organic, there is a living and dying, a precarious ecological balance involving particles in motion.

The transmitters reside in little pockets called *vesicles*, located in each cell's presynaptic-nerve ending. When the transmitters cross the synapse, they land at *receptor sites*, which are molecularly structured to fit particular transmitter families. When enough receptor sites are occupied by transmitters, the cell of those receptors is stimulated to fire. The resulting impulse runs through the nerve and releases new transmitters that pass on to the next cell.

It looks like this:

FIGURE 2

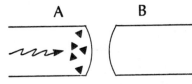

1. An electrical impulse passes through Nerve Cell A.

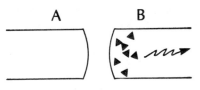

2. When it reaches the end, it releases neurotransmitters into the synapse.

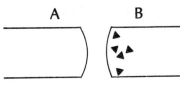

3. The transmitters occupy receptor sites on Nerve Cell B.

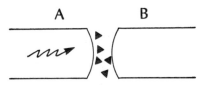

4. When enough receptor sites are occupied, Nerve Cell B begins to fire.

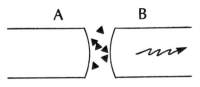

5. When Nerve Cell B fires, the transmitters are released back into the synapse.

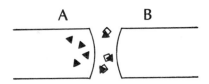

6. Some transmitters are destroyed by enzymes, others return to "home base" in Nerve Cell A.

All this takes place in a thousandth of a second. When the cycle is complete, Nerve Cell A will be ready to fire again.

A moment's reflection makes it apparent that we must have many different kinds of nerve tracts. We have nerves for pain, for glands, for muscle contraction, even for transmitting visual and auditory data. The study of these systems is one of the most complicated subjects in all of medicine. We could fill a dozen volumes with what we know about it, and it would take a hundred more just to say what we don't know.

For simplicity's sake:

Starting at the top of your brain and working down through the nerves in your spinal column, the lower you go the less inhibitory the nerves become, until finally they are nothing more than specialized automatons. You could compare the nervous system with a human society. The decision-making power resides in the "executive branch," but the executive can function only by the grace of the subordinates, including the many laborers whose efforts are rarely recognized.

Our nervous system's executive is the *cortex*. It sits on top of the *central nervous system*. In humans the cortex is highly developed and is responsible for most of our "higher intelligence." The *voluntary nervous system* is the system that operates our motor muscles. It is under the control of the central nervous system, and it is subject to the orders it receives from the consciousness.

Descending still lower, we come to the *autonomic nervous system*. This system flows out through every part of our anatomy. We are rarely, if ever, aware of its functions, since it operates without any conscious volition. The autonomic nervous system falls into two different categories—the *sympathetic nervous system* and the *parasympathetic nervous system*. They work in a kind of competition, like two parallel currents that are constantly controlling each other.

The sympathetic nerves are our bodies' "accelerators." They dilate your pupils, they activate your sweat glands, they speed your heart rate and tighten your sphincters and help bring out feelings of anxiety or aggressiveness.

Parasympathetic nerves are the body's "braking system." They do everything opposite to the sympathetic nerves. They slow your heart rate, increase your speed of digestion and make you feel relaxed and at peace with your surroundings. The equal balance of these two systems creates a feeling of normalcy. Only when one of the systems is inhibited does the other become dominant; we then feel uncomfortable.

There are other important nerve categories. One, the *pyramidal tract*, is actually part of your voluntary nervous system, helping instruct and stimulate many motor activities. Have you ever seen a person who has suffered from a stroke? You may have noticed how often only one side is affected. And possibly you've been told that the side that is paralyzed is on the *opposite* side from where the brain has been damaged. This is because of the pyramidal tract. For some reason not totally clear to science, these nerve chains crisscross below the cortex so that each side of your brain controls the opposite-side body members.

Parallel to this tract is the *extrapyramidal system*, which also figures in body movement. Although you are totally unconscious of its function, this system gives tone and fluidity to all your muscle activities. If you have ever seen a person with Parkinson's disease, you know how jerky his movements become. This is because parkinsonism attacks the extrapyramidal system, imposing a start-and-stop quality on all motor activities.

Understanding the workings of these systems sheds light on the activities of drugs. Just as there are diseases that attack various nerve families, so drugs can also disrupt certain neuronal functions. This is what the labels in your medicine chest call side effects, meaning that the drug will have an effect on more than one division of the nervous system. The drug may be intended to work on your brain, but it may also affect your breathing or your bowel movements.

Each of these nervous systems contains various transmitter families, and it is the activity of these transmitters that regulates the system. The greater the activity, the more "hyper" the nerve tract; the lower the activity, the more powerful the *opposing* nerve tract. If I wanted to dilate a patient's pupils, I could give him a drug that *increased* sympathetic transmitter activity. Conversely, a drug that *decreased* parasympathetic transmitter activity would produce outward results that are very similar.

But pupil dilation is strictly physiological. There is also a link between transmitters and mood processes. We can actually measure mental and mood alterations by the level of activity of various transmitter families. (Note that I do not say that transmitters *cause* these changes. As we shall come to see later, that has not been proven. But we can say with certainty that levels of transmitter activity are indicators of mood swings—and, in some cases, psychosis.)

Depressed states involve at least two relevant transmitter types: One is *serotonin,* and the other is *norepinephrine.* Most antidepressants in use today raise the level of one or both of these transmitter families. This has led to a neat hypothesis: Increase transmitters and you will elevate the spirit; decrease transmitters and you will calm the patient down—either to a state of tranquility or, if the level is too low, to a depressed condition.

Diagrammatically, it looks like this:

FIGURE 3

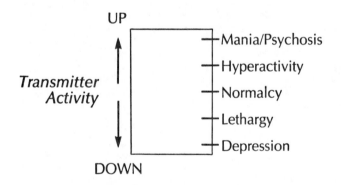

If I had been writing this book ten years ago, I probably would have left you with this pat little formula. We sincerely thought that it was the ultimate answer, and all our new drugs seemed to corroborate its validity. We now suspect that the actual mechanism is much more complicated, but since this theory has been so important to our progress, it is necessary to understand it before you can appreciate its fallacies.

To return to the illustration of you and your spouse at the dinner table, we now have a partially physiological explanation. Something has taken place in the environment that elevated certain transmitter levels and increased your tension. But how can a "thought" have a *physical* effect on you? How can an "idea" elevate transmitter activity? And how is that activity translated into a behavior change—grimacing, trembling, stabbing hostilely at your dinner plate?

To the traditional analyst such phenomena are abstract. They are embraced in concepts like *id* and *guilt complexes*. Some hidden conflict has resulted in anger, producing (by some mysterious means) certain drives and hostilities. Let's say your marriage has been suffering strains of late. You have been secretly resentful of your spouse's working late. Your anger has been triggered by a reference to a co-worker whose name has come up a number of times that month. Is this person a threat? Is your spouse being unfaithful? Or is this only an exposure of your own insecurity? These are the answers an analyst would look for—and indeed they would be helpful in resolving your relationship.

Physiologically, however, these answers are inadequate. They do not explain the true cause and effect. How can an emotion be translated into a hand tremor—particularly when your consciousness is disavowing any knowledge of it?

Viewing this same scene from the perspective of hard science, an abstraction like *jealousy* is not part of the picture. We must reduce such concepts to pure physics and chemistry and follow, as best we can, the chain of activity. All that your spouse has imparted are light waves and sound waves. Not a single "emotion" has crossed the dinner table. There may be intensities of pitch or activity, but these are as devoid of value as radio or television signals.

When these various sense data reach your eyes and ears, they are instantly translated into a series of nerve impulses. The chemicals in your nerve cells create an electrical current, which in turn releases neurotransmitters into the synapse. These impulses are relayed from cell to cell until finally they arrive at some portion of your brain. Your brain decodes them, much like a computer, matching new and stored material on the basis of similarity.

Your brain is programmed to respond to these impulses. The data are transmitted along the loop of the limbic system. The question being asked is whether these data match previous data, and if so, how have we been programmed to respond to them? An answer is found and transmitted to other nerve cells, which, like miniature Paul Reveres, alert your glands and internal organs. Soon you are a virtual cauldron of activity—flushing, tensing, trembling, pulsating.

Meanwhile, has your consciousness ever caught up? Has your cortex been informed of all this activity? Or have inhibitory nerves been brought into play to impede and protect this part of your mental process? We aren't quite sure how this mechanism functions, but it's reasonable to presume that there may be a blocking action. Your body can be literally ravaged by "emotion," while your consciousness remains unable to recognize it.

The sorting and identifying of all these processes is likely to take scientists many, many years. At present the focus is on identifying transmitters and trying to determine their paths of operation. We are also looking for new receptor sites, and the two research projects are interrelated. When we find a new receptor and analyze its structure, it gives us a better idea of what transmitter we're looking for.

This exercise has turned up some tantalizing findings. In 1973 we found our first human "opiate receptors." These are receptor sites in the ends of human brain cells that are molecularly tailored to receive opium and heroin. What, you may ask, are those doing in our heads? Why should our nerve cells be structured for opium? Surely, when Nature laid out the blueprint, she didn't intend for our species to become drug addicts.

Scientists wondered about this, too. We knew those receptors were there for a purpose, so perhaps there was something like opium in our heads which was nonaddictive but worked as a painkiller.

It didn't take long to find the answer. In 1975, at Scotland's

University of Aberdeen, scientists isolated two natural opiates, which they promptly dubbed *enkephalins,* meaning "something in the head." Since then researchers have found still other painkillers, among them *endorphins,* meaning "the morphine within." Still other receptors have been discovered for a variety of substances, including the benzodiazepines like Valium and Librium.

In 1979, at Stanford University, Dr. Avram Goldstein, professor of pharmacology, announced the discovery of our twentieth transmitter, a remarkable substance that Goldstein called *dynorphin.* Dynorphin seems to be an unprecedented painkiller— perhaps two hundred times more powerful than morphine. Yet it is nonaddictive, so if we learn how to use it properly, its benefits could be awesome.

Discoveries like these have led to a host of new miracle drugs, some of which are discussed in later chapters. These drugs result from transmitter research and our increased understanding of our natural brain chemistry. We expect, for example, to produce a successor to Valium. It will be far more potent but produce fewer side effects. Researchers are currently testing chemicals called *purines,* which have a molecular structure that matches our Valium receptors.

Some of these new drugs are already on the market. One is a substance called *naloxone.* It is already in use in hospital emergency rooms, where it is saving the lives of heroin-overdose victims. As might be apparent from the discussion so far, much of our research focuses on addiction. What makes us become so dependent upon one substance, while a similar substance has no marked effect on us? One phenomenon that has fascinated my profession is the discovery of enzymes that break down enkephalins. Apparently we have a family of "detergents" within us that wash away painkillers when we no longer need them. When you inject a rabbit with a lethal dose of morphine, the animal will be at death's door within seconds. The morphine has bound to receptors in the brain that regulate breathing via the central nervous system. When this rabbit is injected with naloxone, however, within seconds the animal will be back on its feet. The naloxone has blocked the action of the morphine. The rabbit acts almost as if nothing had ever happened to it.

The discovery of natural opiates leads to speculation: Is this why our bodies are sometimes immune to pain? Is this why a man can lose a leg in battle and say that he feels absolutely nothing? Do we have other substances for psychic distress? What creates shock during periods of grief? How do some people survive devastating tragedy and continue to function as if nothing has happened to them?

We think natural painkillers are a clue to these phenomena, and we soon expect to be able to match them in a laboratory. This will be a significant achievement, particularly in the fight against situational illnesses.

Some of these discoveries are almost tantamount to wizardry. They have excited researchers and raised expectations. I am afraid that there might now be some psychiatrists who have become attracted to drugs to the detriment of their other functions. If you reexamine that dinner-table scene, it is apparent that there are at least two elements involved—one is what is happening inside your body, and the other is the environment and how it is affecting you. Some see drugs as the answer to everything; but this ignores the fact that there is a problem in your marriage and that until it is solved your body will react to it. It is like giving your child a dose of cold medicine, then sending him back out to play in the rain. As long as there is an environment that affects our bodies, there will still be a need for psychological therapy.

At the end of this chapter, there is a list of known transmitters and a brief description of how they function. You might find it helpful to refer to this list later when we're talking about illnesses and various drug side effects.

At present, however, the most important order of business is to show how drugs affect neurotransmitters. There are three basic mechanisms—three modes of action—that are relevant to all mood-changers from Thorazine to Valium.

Mechanism #1: Blocking of Receptor Sites

When the scientists in France discovered CPZ, they had no idea of its neuronal function. It was only years later, after a great deal of research, that we learned that CPZ impeded certain transmitters' activity.

Receptor sites, as we explained, are the molecular "landing pads" into which transmitters lock after crossing the synapse. Only when enough receptor sites are occupied is a nerve cell triggered to fire its impulse. Drugs like CPZ and other "major tranquilizers" become attached to the receptor sites at the postsynaptic-nerve end. These drugs themselves do not stimulate the nerve cell, but they effectively prevent the transmitters from stimulating it.

It looks like this:

Blocking of Receptor Sites

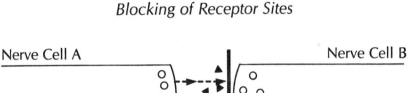

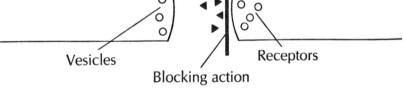

Transmitters travel from Nerve Cell A to Nerve Cell B, where some drugs block them from entering receptors. Brand names of drugs that do this include Thorazine, Stelazine, Mellaril, Haldol, Vesprin, Permitil, Prolixin, Trilafon and Compazine.

In the case of CPZ, one of the transmitters being blocked is a highly important substance in the brain called *dopamine*. An excess of dopamine is associated with schizophrenia, while a deficiency leads to the symptoms of Parkinson's disease. As we shall come to see later, there is a connection between these illnesses, a link that was unearthed by modern drug therapy. CPZ has the effect of *reducing* transmitter activity, and this seems to help in the alleviating of psychosis.

Mechanism #2: Blocking of "Re-uptake"

If the "major tranquilizers" which help schizophrenics lower transmitter activity by blocking the receptors, it is not surprising that the antidepressants have the opposite effect of raising transmitter activity. The method is still a blocking action, only now it is taking place on the *pre*synaptic nerve ending. This means that transmitters cannot return to their vesicles, resulting in an excess of transmitters floating free in the synapse.

Like this:

Blocking of "Re-uptake"

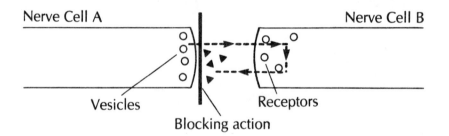

Transmitters go from Nerve Cell A to Nerve Cell B; but on their return trip antidepressants block them from "re-uptake" by vesicles. Brand drugs that do this include Elavil, Tofranil, Aventyl, Sinequan, Adapin, Norpramin, Pertofrane and Vivactil.

The end result is a surplus of transmitters—and, as you would logically assume, more neuronal impulses.

The antidepressants that do this are called *tricyclics*. The transmitters they increase are *serotonin* and *norepinephrine*. The

72

latter is chemically related to adrenaline, so the quickening effect is easy to imagine.

Mechanism #3: Inhibiting Enzymes

There is a third way drugs can affect neurotransmitter activity—by inhibiting enzymes that destroy transmitters. One of these enzymes is *monoamine oxidase* (MAO), which is stored near the vesicles in the presynaptic-nerve ending.

If you refer to the illustration on page 73, you will see that a transmitter's journey is a perilous flight. On its return trip to the vesicles in the presynaptic-nerve cell, it can be destroyed by MAO. This is a natural part of the body's metabolism and, as we shall illustrate later, beneficial. But if you inhibit MAO, you increase the transmitters' survival rate, with the result being greater neuronal activity.

Inhibiting Enzymes

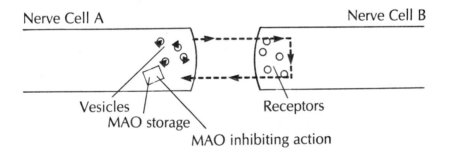

Transmitters travel from Nerve Cell A to Nerve Cell B. On the return trip some would normally be destroyed by MAO. However, MAO inhibitors whose US brands include Marplan, Nardil, Eutonyl and Parnate block MAO from destroying the neurotransmitters.

The drugs with this activity are called *MAO inhibitors*. Like tricyclics, they are antidepressants. They, too, work on serotonin and norepinephrine, the neurotransmitters most linked with depressed states.

I cautioned earlier against leaping to the conclusion that transmitter activity actually *causes* mood change. For scientists the connection is purely associative, but it is a useful connection for tailoring pharmaceuticals. If we learn that a drug lowers the level of dopamine, we presume that it might help alleviate psychosis. If another drug raises serotonin or norepinephrine, we check to see if it is helpful for depressed patients. One of the problems we encounter, however, is that the nerves being affected occur throughout the body. The cells we are aiming for are in the brain, but the nerve cells we affect might be in the liver or pancreas.

When you administer a drug to a depressed or psychotic patient, you give the person a pill or, less frequently, an injection. Either way, the drug permeates the body, affecting every transmitter for which it has an affinity. Pills cause an additional problem because they enter the body through the stomach, where much of their efficacy is destroyed by enzymes. The amount available for delivery to the brain is a relatively small fraction of the original quantity.

To complicate matters, surrounding the brain is a thicket of capillaries called the *blood-brain barrier*. Any substance that tries to penetrate this barrier soon becomes dissipated in a maze of alleyways. This makes drug taking a wasteful proposition. Only 2 percent may be getting through the barrier. Ninety-eight percent may be affecting other areas, creating a host of side effects from dry mouth to heart failure.

Finding ways to foil the blood-brain barrier has become a major priority in psychopharmacology. The more of a drug we can slip past these capillaries, the less there will be to pollute our other organs. There are a number of solutions being bandied about. Some doctors suggest that we should change our "delivery system"—that we should inject mood changers through arteries in the neck, or use pinpoint X-rays to penetrate the blood-brain barrier.

Dr. Leo E. Hollister of Stanford University, who has given this subject a good bit of thought, has suggested that we might alter a drug's molecules so that it will seek out specific locations in the brain. We don't have the means of doing this right now, but there might be a clue in certain substances, called *precursors,* which are partially built biochemicals that are on their way to developing into neurotransmitters.

One precursor you may have heard about is a substance called *L-dopa,* which is used to treat parkinsonism. L-dopa is a building block of the transmitter dopamine, which seems to be a factor in both schizophrenia and parkinsonism. Treating parkinsonism requires added levels of dopamine, but dopamine does not penetrate the blood-brain barrier. L-dopa, on the other hand, does pass through. When it enters the brain, it is converted to dopamine.

To give you an example of the complexities of this science: I mentioned earlier monoamine oxidase (MAO). This neuronal substance seems to contribute to depression by destroying transmitters such as serotonin and norepinephrine. We can inhibit MAO through MAO inhibitors, enabling these transmitters to increase and multiply. Unfortunately, since the inhibiting action takes place throughout the body, there can be dangerous side effects and, in rare cases, fatality.

Lately we have discovered that even MAO comes in a variety of molecular configurations. The MAO in the liver, for example, is not quite the same as the MAO in brain cells. If we can devise a drug—and I'm sure someone is working on it—that only inhibits the MAO in our brains, we can conceivably treat a patient for depression without having to worry about what else we may be doing.

Still another way we are hoping to improve drugs is by using them with peripherally inhibiting molecules—that is, molecules that will let the drug pass to the target area but block its activities on other parts of the body. The hypothesis is that if a drug is frustrated from entering areas not relevant to therapy, it will remain free to float through the vascular system until, for want of other avenues, it will enter the brain cells. This, too, has been achieved in the treatment of Parkinson's disease. We can administer L-dopa with a substance called *carbidopa*. The carbidopa stops L-dopa from turning into dopamine except in the brain area, where such conversion is desirable.

This gives you an overview of the basic principles. It does not equip you to become a psychopharmacologist, but it provides you with the pegs on which to hang the research that our profession now applies to certain illnesses. Those illnesses are the subject of the next few chapters. We'll begin with depression and go on to cover everything from mania to phobia to anxiety, including that most terrifying of diseases, schizophrenia.

In the meantime I would like to leave you with some thoughts that have become axiomatic among psychopharmacologists. I think they are valid generalizations, although, as in most of life, there may be exceptions.

1. All behavior has a chemical component. This is as true of our mental as it is of our physical behavior. While *what* we think may have extraordinary value, our *mechanism* of thinking is physiological.

2. All mental illness is psychosomatic—or *somatopsychic*. The process may start either in our bodies or in our environment, but the illness is physical and can be measured empirically. This gives the lie to that stigma called madness. There is nothing imaginary about an illness that strikes your body.

3. We can measure our emotions through neurotransmitters, which act as messengers between the cells in our nerve tracts. Everything we do, everything we think, seems to affect and be affected by our neurotransmitters.

4. The mood-changing drugs most psychiatrists now prescribe are designed to work on a person's neurotransmitters. Their effect is medical—they are in no way magical—and there is massive research behind every one of them. Moreover, these new drugs are designed to cure illness. They will not make a normal person feel any happier. In fact, most normal people are affected adversely by them, which makes them virtually useless as "street drugs."

5. Finally, all drugs still have unwanted side effects, arising from activities in other parts of your body. We have reason to believe that the drugs of tomorrow will show considerable improvement in this troublesome area.

FIGURE 4
Some Neurotransmitters and How They Affect You

Neuro-Transmitter	Location	Increased level	Decreased level
Norepinephrine (also called nor-adrenaline)	central nervous system; sympathetic nerves throughout the body	hyperactivity and stress; high blood pressure; increased breathing capacity; constipation; relaxation of bladder; dilation of pupils	depression; constriction of lungs; diarrhea; contracted pupils.
Acetylcholine	brain; parasympathetic nerves throughout body	lethargy; increased salivation; slowing of heart-rate; contraction of pupils, bladder and bowels	muscle weakness or paralysis; hallucination; disorientation and agitation
Dopamine	brain; central nervous system	schizophrenia; mania; hallucinations	Parkinson's disease; jerky body movements; depression (?)
Serotonin	brain; central nervous system	hallucinations and increased sleep	depression; insomnia; aggression; hypersexual behavior

Histamine	throughout body	dilation of blood vessels; puffiness; itching; in central nervous system, depression (?)	in central nervous system, perhaps antidepressant effect
GABA	brain and spinal cord	relaxation; Valium-like effects	parkinsonism (?); schizophrenia (?); Alzheimer's disease (?)
Enkephalins	brain	deadening of pain	narcotic withdrawal symptoms
Endorphins	pituitary gland; brain	deadening of pain	narcotic withdrawal symptoms

5

Depression—Of Cheddar Cheese and Darwin

There's a theory making the rounds in psychiatry that depression may be linked to evolution—that is, it may be part of an adaptive process to promote and secure the preservation of our species.

How, one might ask, does science arrive at this? Evolution is a positive, depression is a negative. That there might be a connection between the two seems improbable at best, at worst an absurdity.

Consider:

Depression is hardly new to humanity—it is one of the oldest complaints of civilization. The ancient Greeks were very concerned about it, and it was pondered by everyone from Homer to Aristotle. In *The Anatomy of Melancholy*, Robert Burton, in seventeenth-century England, seemed to speak for his era as he pondered the enigma of this most troublesome malady:

> I'll change my state with any wretch
> Thou canst from gaol or dunghill fetch.
> My pain's past cure, another Hell,

I may not in this torment dwell.
Now desperate I hate my life,
Lend me a halter or a knife.
  All my griefs to this are jolly
  Naught so damned as Melancholy.

Burton probably didn't realize it, but he was onto something very important: namely, that depression seems to have a plaguelike quality that leaves its mark on a whole society. Post-Elizabethan England was one such period. The Romantic period was probably another. In the hands of such poets as Keats and Shelley, depression becomes an art form.

Evidence suggests that we are in another such era, although we seem to lack the poets to give it voice and resonance. Rather, it shows up in the faces of the patients who occupy the seats in my waiting room. Thirty years ago we were in the Age of Anxiety. We fought it with barbiturates, Miltown and Equanil. Today we have returned to an Age of Depression, and you can see it reflected on every psychiatrist's prescription pad.

Why this is so is a matter of conjecture. Perhaps our hopes have outstripped all reality. Our age abounds with promises of fulfillment that never quite match the true situation. Presidents promise Great Societies, and instead we are torn by war and conflict. As our salaries increase, so do prices and taxes, and we find ourselves pinched by the earth's dwindling resources. There is even a "hope gap" in our personal and sex lives. We seek pleasure and ecstasy, and we are rewarded with boredom. Justice and perfection remain will-o'-the-wisps, and our souls grow sour in the futile pursuit.

If society itself is a kind of organism, then it makes sense that a society might suffer such reactions. They are a natural reflex, a conditioned response not unlike what happens when we inhibit a nervous system. "Slow down," we seem to be saying to ourselves. "We are letting our dreams get ahead of our capacities. Relax. Go to sleep. Take a forced retirement. As unpleasant as it seems, in the long run you'll be better for it."

This, of course, is just sociological wool gathering, but there is some hard evidence that depression may be a tool—that in its purest state, unencumbered by symbolism, it is a means of saving more lives than it destroys. Some impressive studies conducted during the past ten years have shown that animals, like humans, also suffer from depression. Behaviorally and physiologically their reactions to this illness are not unlike the reactions of infants and young people. If you take a small animal away from its mother, its first expression will be rage and protest. After that the animal will become asocial and withdrawn, showing all the signs of clinical depression. The theory is that this may be a signal that alerts other animals that this young one is in trouble. When human children act in similar fashion, we feel an instinctive desire to give aid and support to them.

The problem is that as we humans get older, we develop a penchant for frustrating nature. What in children may be an appropriate response becomes inappropriate, or self-destructive, in adults. The loss of a mother is a genuine threat to a child. If he does not sound an alarm, the child is in danger of perishing. When screaming doesn't help, there is no better distress signal than to become indolent, lethargic and unresponsive to his social group. As we grow older, "Mother" grows complicated. We begin to crowd her presence with symbols and surrogates. Eventually the symbols replace the original, and we get depressed over things that have no crucial meaning to us. Will we die, for example, if a lover walks out on us? Does it threaten our lives when we are denied a promotion? No, these are simply disappointments to which we may find ourselves reacting with a primitive magnitude.

In psychiatry we don't like to use the word *depression*. We prefer using phrases like *affective disorder*. This, of course, is professional jargon, but it does serve a purpose among those who are semantics oriented. You'll recall that we said the limbic system is the area in the brain where our moods originate. We attach emotion to various thoughts and images, which until then had been valueless—just pure, raw sense data. Among psychiatric disorders there are two basic categories—those that disrupt thought and those that disrupt mood. To the former belong illnesses like schizophrenia, in which the thought processes become confused and hallucinatory.

Depression, however, is a mood disorder. *Affect* is simply a synonym for *mood*. Depressed people usually have fairly clear thought processes. They don't see pink elephants, and they don't hear voices. The problem is that they take logical thoughts and attach them to emotions that are consistently self-derogatory. If you were to say to a depressed person, "I can't see you tomorrow night," he is likely instantly to construct this to mean that you don't like him. It will confirm his suspicion that he is loathsome and inferior, and no matter how hard you try, you will not fully dissuade him of that.

Freud, of course, defined depression as hostility that has been redirected inward. This is valid, at least psychoanalytically, and none of our findings should be viewed as contradicting it. In other words, when someone hurts us, and that someone is beyond our appropriate anger, we take our hostility and direct it inward, offering ourselves as available scapegoats. Certainly we have all known depressed people who do that. A spouse dies suddenly, and the widow or widower feels deserted. But who is there to blame? The person has no one to strike out at and so may beat himself into a slough of despondency.

The essential problem with the Freudian theory is that it fails to recognize different *kinds* of depression. Freud assumed that all depression was triggered by experience—although, as reserpine showed us, some causes are chemical. Reserpine, you'll recall from the discussion on page 33, was the Rauwolfia extract that deprived high blood pressure patients of their motivation. This indicated a biological problem that had nothing to do with hostility or guilt feelings.

In the stratum of psychiatry called *nosology*—the classification of various illnesses—depression has been broken down into two distinct categories, each with its own presumed causes and origins. One type of depression has been called *reactive depression*. This comes as a response to an outside event. It can be described as a sadness which doesn't debilitate or incapacitate.

For *endogenous depression*, however, there may be no discernible cause. It may come and go, cyclic, mysterious. It is more serious, more implacable, more paralyzing, striking again and again without justification. The majority of research in recent years has been directed to this kind of biological illness. One reason for this is that the drugs we have discovered seem to work best against endogenous depression.

But the distinction between these definitions is blurred. Events that can make us unhappy occur with every tick of the clock. In the majority of cases an interim of grief is inevitably followed by a return to normalcy. What makes one person overreact? Why does he flounder in such bottomless gloom? Are we to assume that just because the origin is obvious, the resultant disorder is any less perilous?

The trail of this reasoning leads us back to the laboratory. Is there an agent in these people that makes them so vulnerable? Is there a substance or hormone—or perhaps a lack of one—that impedes or prevents emotional recovery? I wish I could give you an easy answer to that, but even the answers we do have are often conjectural. But we have found certain approaches, or models, that may open the door to vastly improved therapies.

The Predrug Approach

When you go to a psychiatrist complaining of depression, she does not start off by giving you a pill. Following the traditional analyst's approach, she begins by asking you a series of questions that are designed to clarify the exact nature of your complaint. Our notions of depression as a nonmedical phenomenon are still well rooted in Freudian concepts. We see depression as a force or drive that has become misdirected and, as a result, self-punitive.

Since Freud this idea has gained some refinements. Freud placed great emphasis on early childhood. He viewed depression as transformed hostility whose roots could be traced to a need for nurturing. Like most of Freud's theories, his view of depression has proved quite durable against the onslaught of skepticism, but a more recent theory has downplayed the importance of childhood events and considered depression as an evolutionary defense mechanism.

Recently the cognitive theory has begun to emerge. This theory claims that, though depression is a mood disorder, its origins may be rooted in thought processes irrespective of biochemical factors. You'll recall the anecdote about the man at the dinner table: His problem was twofold—it was both chemical and psychic. While we could show the physical effect on his nervous system, that did not negate a psychological conflict. Psychopharmacology does not contradict other therapies. We still search for patterns in people's behavior and thought processes. To reduce all life to a study of transmitters would not only be boring, it would be superficial.

In the cognitive view each person has a schema—a pattern or bias with which he or she views life—and this is what determines that person's responses, so that even moods are the pawns of an individual's outlook. People who have a tendency toward depression have schemas concerned with self-deprecation. Those who develop anxiety states have schemas that anticipate personal injury.

There is evidence that depressed people *think* differently, and also that what they *do* think is colored by their mood processes. But how can we determine which disturbance is primary? Even if there is a difference in thought patterns, how do we know that moods weren't responsible, working backward, as it were, through a kind of Pavlovian conditioning process?

Nevertheless, I think this theory has merit. Indeed, it has been valuable in helping some depressed patients. Dr. Aaron Beck at the University of Pennsylvania has become a leading advocate of cognitive-therapy programs.

Perhaps here it is appropriate to define exactly what we mean by *depression*. Depression is *not* the same as unhappiness, and from a psychiatric standpoint it is important to distinguish between the two. If you go to a doctor saying that you are depressed, that you are extremely unhappy with your lot in life, that you find yourself erupting into unexplained crying jags and you don't feel like working or getting up in the morning—this is not proof that you are actually depressed. Rather, these are signs that you are only unhappy. Your unhappiness may or may not be well founded, but it will not be alleviated by tricyclics or other chemicals. *True depression is manifested as a physical illness.* It has certain signs that we call *vegetative symptoms*. These include insomnia, weight loss and the inability to perceive pleasure. They are of central importance for diagnosis. Of course, there are many gradations of depression, just as there are for other illnesses, but *unless you have the "vegetative symptoms," no reputable physician will put you on drug therapy.*

Many physicians make a diagnosis on the basis of certain innocent-seeming questions. If the patient answers the questions honestly, it helps us define the nature of the problem:

Are you able to experience pleasure in anything?

Do you view your past as being happier than your present?

Do you have a dread of getting up in the morning?

Do you enjoy eating, or does your food taste flat? Do you notice any unusual change in appetite?

Do you have trouble getting to sleep at night? Conversely, do you wake up too early in the morning? Have you noticed any appreciable change in sleep patterns, such as sleeping too late or taking naps during the daytime?

Do you find it hard to concentrate at work?

Do you find it difficult to read a book?

Have you noticed any unusual slowdown in activity? Are you spending more time in front of the television?

Have you ever thought of taking your own life? If so, when? Within the past few days? Were there other times when you thought about suicide? Did you ever make plans as to how you would accomplish it?

Have you had unusual trouble remembering things lately?

Do you find that everyday tasks seem more burdensome and difficult?

Would you characterize your future as being meaningless or hopeless?

Have you experienced an unusual disinterest in sex lately?

To these behavioral questions, one might add medically oriented questions. Have you lost weight lately? Are your bowel movements normal? Have you had dizziness? Dry mouth? An irregular menstrual cycle?

We know from many years of experience that too many yes answers are a sign of depression. Many patients will not even know they're depressed, only that they have insomnia and are having trouble functioning. Of course the patient could have another illness, some disease or malady that has gone undetected. A good physician will be aware of this possibility and may insist that the patient undergo medical tests.

Having determined that the problem is depression, the doctor will now determine the *kind* of depression. Has it happened before? Is it a cyclical illness? Or is there a recent event that seems to have traumatized the psyche? (Let me stress here that the order of these questions is purely arbitrary and may vary with circumstances. Indeed, many fine doctors simply begin their questioning with the bald remark, "Do you feel depressed?") In order to determine endogenous depression, the doctor will ask for a family history. Was your mother depressed? Was your dad an alcoholic? Were any of your relatives unstable or suicidal? As will become apparent later, this is important information. There is very strong evidence that depression can be hereditary. From a treatment standpoint the doctor is clued that the causes of the illness may be biochemical.

The doctor will now consider possible courses. Should one prescribe a drug or recommend analysis? The current trend is to opt for the drug, though often in conjunction with psychotherapy. But if the doctor chooses a drug, what drug should it be? There are approximately a dozen different antidepressants.

How do they work? What do they do to you? And, most important, which is apt to work best for you?

In Chapter 4, in our discussion of transmitters, we explained the activity of certain antidepressants. We showed how, by a couple of simple mechanisms, they increased the activity along certain nerve tracts. But to understand the complexity of the problem and the variety of treatments under consideration, we must first take a look at the chemical approaches, which at the present fall into three general categories.

The Neurotransmitter Approach

As I mentioned in Chapter 4, our moods seem linked to certain transmitter activity. When these transmitters hop faster, our mood goes up; when their activity declines, we slip into depression. I use the words *seem linked* not because we have doubts about this but because there are questions we have yet to find answers for. What, for example, causes manic-depression, in which both highs and lows come out of the same neurochemical system?

The evidence in support of the neurotransmitter theory is mostly founded on our research in drugs. We know, for example, that a drug like reserpine will deplete neurotransmitters and create feelings of depression. Conversely, there are other drugs that increase neurotransmitters and produce alertness, frenzy and hyperactivity. That there is some sort of link between transmitters and mood seems too well established to be coincidental.

One of the chief suspects as an instigator of depression is the neurotransmitter *norepinephrine*. This is found in the central nervous system and in sympathetic nerve tracts throughout the body. A depletion of norepinephrine levels leads to a number of behavioral and biological changes. Heart rate slows, pupils contract, a person becomes lethargic, asocial and doesn't feel like doing anything.

Serotonin, which is found in the brain, is another neurotransmitter receiving a lot of attention. Evidence shows that a disturbance in this substance may contribute to depression in a large number of patients. One of the ways we can replenish

88

serotonin is by administering an amino acid called *tryptophan*. Tryptophan, which is found in many plants and animals, is a precursor, or building block, of serotonin. There is evidence that tryptophan may be particularly effective for the part of depression that disrupts sleep patterns. It is still one of the paradoxes of this complicated science that a drug that lifts your spirits will also help you sleep better.

Most of the drugs we use to fight depression are both derived from and supportive of the neurotransmitter theory. Using them, we can achieve cure rates of 70 percent or better, depending upon the drug and the severity of the illness. Among these drugs are tricyclic antidepressants, MAO inhibitors, lithium and tryptophan. Occasionally they are used in combination, or in combination with other drugs such as a tranquilizing agent.

Another treatment that we use to fight depression, and which corroborates our theories about neurotransmitters, is ECT— electroconvulsive therapy—the oldest and most potent of our depression combatants. You may recall, when I was talking about the early days of drugs, that I said that my training had been primarily Freudian. Yet I had seen firsthand the effects of electroshock, and I had long been curious about the biological why of it. This may strike some people as a rather crude line of research; indeed, some of my colleagues were very disapproving. I remember one day being called aside by a superior, who warned me sternly not to become a "button-pusher"!

Yet, I had two very good reasons for my interest in electroshock. One was that I had always had an interest in chemistry. The other was that I could see that electroshock *worked!* It was doing more to help depressed patients than all our hours of analysis.

Depression, unlike other maladies, strikes people who are normal and brings them to their knees. Executives, family people, grandmothers, college students—one day they're happy and the next they're miserable. In a schizophrenic the change is not so dramatic. There's often been a history of withdrawn behavior. But you can *relate* to a depressive. You can see that he is like you. And when you heal him, it's like being a witness to a miracle.

But there we were, locked in our ignorance, surrounded by the notions of false humanitarianism, refusing to provide the one cure we had because it didn't fit the concepts of abstract analysis. Were we healers or weren't we? When psychotropic drugs arrived I jumped at the opportunity to apply for grants to do research on electroshock.

As a scientist, I knew that the laws of electricity were practically inseparable from the laws of chemistry. We were talking about atoms—the flow of electrons—and this obviously would have an effect on biology. Indeed, the earliest shock treatments were performed with chemicals. Shock by electricity is relatively recent. Previously, substances like insulin and camphor had been used to create the same convulsions with similar effectiveness.

My earliest experiments were on the effects of ECT and the changes it caused in the blood-brain barrier. Many of the findings have since been refined. We now have several hypotheses as to why ECT helps people.

I am discussing ECT in a book devoted to drug therapy because ECT remains a common remedy. A person suffering from severe depression should not be frightened if the doctor suggests a series of shock treatments. The doctor should not suggest this unless the case is severe. The doctor should also be convinced that, with other therapy, the risk to the patient would be unacceptable.

I'll illustrate with a hypothetical case: Say I receive a phone call from a terrified woman. Her husband, whom I have been treating for depression, has become so despondent that he has just tried to hang himself. I hastily arrange an emergency meeting with him. When he arrives, I find that he is in severe depression. His despair is so deep that he can hardly function. He has now reached the point where only death seems sensible to him.

This man is a candidate for ECT. I have already tried a drug, and the drug isn't working. Were I to change his prescription, it would take weeks of readjustment, and I would have no guarantee of the new drug's efficacy. The cure rate for drugs is in the 70 to 80 percent range (that's against a cure rate for placebos of about 20 to 30 percent), whereas the cure rate for shock is better than 90 percent, a significant odds increase in the face of such morbidity.

The most significant factor is the time element. This man has shown clearly that he is at the end of the line. "Whatever you do, it had better be fast," he is saying, "because I have no intention of enduring this hell that I'm suffering." Shock, of course, is frightening to most patients. They equate electricity with light sockets and electric chairs. It seems inconceivable to them that it can also be beneficial. Some persuasion is often necessary to get them to sign a release form.

At this point one is faced with an ethical dilemma—the patient's right to die versus the doctor's duty to save him. I am not God, I cannot sit in judgment; but I have a responsibility both to myself and to this man's loved ones. I would not recommend shock were there another way, simply because the idea so frightens people. We are conditioned to popping little pills out of bottles, but not to being treated by a jolt out of a generator.

The media have done little to allay these fears. We equate ECT with something horrible, dehumanizing. We see movies like *The Snake Pit* or *One Flew Over the Cuckoo's Nest*, and electroconvulsive therapy looks like medically sanctioned sadomasochism. We also live with the taint of our own past failures: the dung-gray institutions, the horror of straightjackets, the psychosurgery fad of the early 1950s in which more than fifty thousand patients were lobotomized with icepicks. It is no wonder that patients are afraid, since we have done little to improve the image of ECT. Actually modern ECT is a very humane treatment, perhaps in some ways less dangerous than some of our drug treatments.

There is nothing mysterious about the employment of electricity. We *are* electricity. It is in every nerve cell. Shock, like drugs, stimulates neural activity. It also affects the blood-brain barrier, creating a freer access for various of our body substances.

But the good news is our technical advancement. Today's shock treatments are painless and nonfrightening. Convulsions are nonexistent, there is little memory loss and the whole thing is over in a couple of seconds. This is attributable to several advances. First of all, we now use general anesthesia. This means that the patient is totally unconscious and experiences little apprehension concerning the mechanics of the physical procedure.

Second, we use a chemical called *succinylcholine*, which completely eliminates peripheral convulsions. The only effect is on the central nervous system. There is no spasm or thrashing of the extremities.

Finally—and this is only since 1957—we no longer stimulate both lobes of the brain. We now use what is called a *unilateral stimulus,* in which the charge only goes through the nondominant temporal lobe. This, we have found, cuts the amount of memory loss. In the old days some patients suffered significant amnesia. Today a person can come in for a shock treatment and be back in the office within twenty-four hours.

In fairness, we still have some questions about shock. Might it cause minimal damage to the blood-brain barrier? Is there any evidence that the average shock patient may suffer deterioration of perceptual or motor abilities? The overwhelming evidence supports the safety of shock treatment and suggests that its benefits far outweigh its liabilities. An oft-neglected truth is that medicine involves risk. There is a risk to removing a tumor or an appendix. In the end the patient must decide whether the risk is worth the alternative consequences. In psychiatry, of course, this question is compounded because the patient may not be in complete control of himself. We may have to turn to his friends and loved ones to seek a rounded judgment of all the factors involved.

In certain extreme cases, where time and efficacy are crucial, I would urge the patient to undergo shock treatment, then I would administer antidepressants to sustain him in an emotional "holding pattern." Such cases do not have to involve attempted suicide. The patient may have a job that requires quick therapy. He may be a judge or a politician, whose continued depression might have widespread consequences. In psychiatry we treat all kinds of people. I have treated surgeons in whose hands rest lives. Should I tell such a person, "Well, just keep on functioning, and I'm sure in a few months we'll all look back and laugh at this."

Psychiatry remains more than just chemicals and test tubes. It encompasses a wide range of extenuating circumstances. It requires careful listening and a delicacy of judgment, and that is not something that can be taught in either a textbook or a laboratory.

*   *   *

Short of recommending ECT, a doctor's first choice of therapy is likely to be drugs. He may administer them in conjunction with analysis or some other program to help the patient cope better. The drugs the doctor prescribes will fall into one of three categories: They will either be tricyclics, MAO inhibitors or, if there is mania involved, lithium. Most doctors prefer to start with tricyclics, which are easier to use and have a very high cure rate. The illustration on page 72 shows how tricyclics increase transmitters by blocking "re-uptake."

Tricyclics encompass a number of derivatives, but the parent is a compound called *imipramine*. In the United States this is marketed under the trade name Tofranil, whose cousins include Elavil and a half-dozen other substances. Imipramine was discovered in 1958 by Dr. Roland Kuhn and a group of Swiss scientists. They had originally been searching for a sleeping pill— but, as in so many drug stories, ignorance proved fortuitous.

We call this family of drugs tricyclics because its chemical structure contains three connected hydrocarbon rings. It is chemically effective on endogenous depression when the patient is lethargic, withdrawn and indolent. The patient on tricyclics may experience certain side effects, such as dry mouth, constipation, palpitations and dizziness. He may also suffer from headaches, blurred vision and a variety of other minor nuisances. People with glaucoma and people with prostate conditions must be careful of this drug. It can also cause problems among elderly patients, who may suffer more acutely from some of the already-mentioned symptoms.

If the tricyclic drugs don't seem to work—and it will take several weeks to find that out—the doctor may prescribe an MAO inhibitor, which is a little more involved but, at least technically, interesting.

Tricyclics increase neurotransmitters by blocking their return to the presynaptic nerve ending. This raises the level of neurotransmitters floating around in the synaptic space. Transmitter activity can also be increased by inhibiting the enzyme that destroys neurotransmitters. The name of this enzyme is *monoamine oxidase*, which researchers have shortened to MAO.

The history of MAO inhibitors is one of the most fascinating stories in psychopharmacology. Once again, MAO was discovered by accident, having originally been used to treat tuberculosis. Soon doctors discovered that something was wrong: some depressed tubercular patients became entirely too happy! They would overextend themselves, get involved in activities, often ignore the physician's precautions.

Riding the crest of the excitement created by reserpine, Dr. Nathan S. Kline was first on the scene. He reasoned that if reserpine could calm people down, a drug like this might have the reverse effect. He took an inhibitor with the brand name Marsilid and tested it on a group of twenty depressed women. Five weeks later he began to see results—70 percent of the patients showed definite improvement.

But MAO inhibitors contained other surprises, and they have taught us a valuable lesson about the importance of side effects. They have also shown the connection between diet and drugs and how everything we ingest interacts with everything else.

In 1963, in the British medical journal *Lancet,* a distinguished physician named Barry Blackwell published a review of twelve cases of cerebral hemorrhage that had occurred among patients on MAO inhibitors. Nobody saw any connection at the time. We knew that these drugs inhibited monoamine oxidase, but we didn't know why that would cause such a side effect. A hospital pharmacist named G.E.F. Rowe happened to read the article and wrote a letter to Blackwell. His wife, he said, had had a high blood pressure episode, and she too was on an MAO inhibitor. He went on to say that this incident had happened right after his wife had eaten some cheese. He wondered if the hypertension she had suffered could be traced to some substance in the cheddar cheese.

Blackwell and his associates had a good laugh at that. Why would cheese create cerebral hemorrhage? There was no known connection between cheese and MAO inhibitors, and the whole thing was dismissed as utter coincidence.

But at about that time a traveling drug salesman paid a call on Blackwell and made the same observation: His company had received two letters from physicians describing similar incidents among some of their patients. Blackwell began to take more notice. He reviewed the dietary history of two such cases: One was a man who had died while on the drug, and the other was a woman who had experienced an upsurge of blood pressure. Both had eaten cheese.

About this time, in a seemingly unrelated study, another scientist named Milne reported that the intake of Gorgonzola cheese led to the appearance in the blood of a substance called tyramine. Tyramine is a substance which can increase blood pressure and is found in many foods we eat. What we didn't know, and what we only learned later, was that it was normally destroyed by the MAO inside us!

So now we had stumbled across an astounding piece of knowledge: MAO inhibitors blocked one of nature's own antidotes. If you took this drug you could become sick, even die, if you combined it with a food containing the amino acid tyramine. At first this created a shock wave in the industry, and the FDA took precautionary steps. Later the risks were determined to be very small. Now there are a number of companies producing MAO inhibitors. When a doctor prescribes an MAO inhibitor, it is accompanied by a list containing substances to avoid. The chances of problems occurring are only one in thousands, but the patient is advised to follow those instructions. Among the substances are:

avocado	sour cream
caviar	soy sauce
cheeses (aged)	yeast
chianti wine	yogurt
chocolate	allergy pills
chicken liver	decongestants
pickled herring	diet pills
pods of broad beans	nasal sprays

I mentioned earlier an agent called tryptophan. Occasionally a doctor may prescribe this for depression. It seems to alleviate some depression, and there is evidence that it helps snap insomnia cycles. Tryptophan is found in many living organisms, but the tryptophan we use is an extract of turkey glands. Tryptophan administered with an MAO inhibitor has been suggested to be an effective antidepressant.

All chemical remedies have one thing in common: They all have an effect on certain neurotransmitters. Here is a list of antidepressants by brand, so that you can match trade names with their chemical activities.

Antidepressants

Generic Name	Brand Name	Company
Tricyclics		
amitriptyline	Elavil	Merck
desipramine	Pertofrane	USV
	Norpramin	Pharmaceutical, Geigy Lakeside
imipramine	Tofranil	Geigy
nortriptyline	Aventyl	Lilly
protriptyline	Vivactil	Merck
trimipramine	Surmontil	Rhone-Poulenc
doxepin	Sinequan	Pfizer/Roerig
Tetracyclics		
maprotiline	Ludiomil	Ciba
MAO Inhibitors		
isocarboxazid	Marplan	Roche
phenelzine	Nardil	Warner
tranylcypromine	Parnate	Smith, Kline & French

But affecting neurotransmitters is only one of our approaches. Scientists are looking at other avenues, which may turn out to have profound significance.

The Endocrine Approach

Closely allied with the activity of neurotransmitters are the effects of these substances on glands throughout our body. Does our neural activity create depression, or is depression the result of our neurally triggered adrenal system? To some this may sound like the chicken-or-the-egg question—and, indeed, at this point in science it is—but it could be significant if we were eventually to discover that our glands, not our nerves, are the cause of this malady. This would mean, from the standpoint of pharmacology, that we have been doing our repairs on the wrong stretch of track. We could tailor our drugs to work directly on the glandular system and not worry so much about the wiring that fires that system.

My own suspicion is that science will eventually discover that depression is not one neat disease. Like cancer, it is probably a group of diseases that manifest themselves in a few common symptoms. This could be true of all mental disorders. We may find eventually that there are hundreds of causes, but that there are only so many ways a human can behave, so that the symptoms present a deceptive commonality.

At present the endocrine approach to depression does not seem as promising as the transmitter approach. Scientific hypotheses seem to run in fads. This year's fashion becomes next year's attic adornment. As the transmitter hypothesis encounters an increase in skepticism, researchers will be tempted to seek new directions. One of these directions may involve our glands and the myriad substances they pour into the biosystem.

A number of nerve tracts containing neurotransmitters lead to and regulate the hypothalamus, which in turn regulates the pituitary gland, the master gland for a number of other glands.

One of the activities the pituitary gland regulates is the secretion of substances called *corticosteroids*. You've probably heard of the drug group called steroids, which have caused so much controversy among athletes and in betting circles. One corticosteroid is a chemical called *cortisol*, which under normal conditions performs a number of miracles, influencing many metabolic processes and helping us resist things that might otherwise be fatal to us.

We have found that in a number of severely depressed patients, the production of cortisol seems to have run amok. They keep secreting it, even during inactivity, when they are at rest or at night during sleeping hours. Interestingly, this only occurs in *some* depressed patients. We rarely see it in manic-depressives. The people who overproduce cortisol seem to be markedly anxious and are frequently those who contemplate suicide.

We don't know yet what to make of these findings, because we cannot pinpoint where the problem might reside. It might be in the pituitary or in the hypothalamus or in one of the hormones or transmitters that regulate them. Our best guess right now is that the problem will probably lead back to a transmitter malfunction. It is another area we are actively exploring, which may lead to new kinds of chemotherapy.

Two other hormones that may be involved in depression are the growth hormone (GH) and the luteinizing hormone (LH). The first has to do with low blood sugar, the second with women's menses and menopause. In a later chapter we'll discuss hypoglycemia and the role of blood sugar in mental disorders. For now we'll simply mention that GH appears low in some depressed patients who are hypoglycemic.

The hormone LH, which is also transmitter regulated, rises markedly in women after the age of menopause. But a study showed that in depressed women aged fifty-seven to sixty, LH levels were significantly lower. We're not too sure exactly what this means. We know that LH rises in the absence of estrogen. We also know that we can inhibit this rise by reducing the activity of certain of our brain receptors. Since hormones are usually linked to sex drive, the LH findings suggest other avenues—namely that there could be some hormonal dysfunction that is responsible for the lack of libido in depressed patients.

The Electrolyte Approach

In Chapter 4, The Psychic Tennis Game, we showed how electricity passes through a nerve cell, after being created by the action of sodium and potassium, interchanging through a semi-permeable membrane. Sodium and potassium are called *electrolytes*. These are substances that, when placed in solution, become dissociated into ions and are capable of carrying an electrical impulse.

There is some evidence that sodium and potassium may themselves play a role in some forms of depression. As in all of biology, there must be a balance. If the balance is upset, things tend to go haywire. In the illustration on page 62, sodium is outside the membrane and potassium is inside. There is evidence among certain depressed and manic patients that too much sodium is on the inside of the membrane.

What this suggests is that, at least among some manic patients, the entire nerve cell may be overexcitable. As in an unstable compound such as nitroglycerine, there is the constant threat of detonation. As we know, whenever firing occurs, neurotransmitters are released into the synapse. But it may be that in some illnesses this is the *effect*, not the *cause*. The problem may lie in the imbalance of these electrolytes.

We do have a drug that modifies electrolytes—lithium, Dr. John Cade's "miracle." Unfortunately, lithium changes so many other mechanisms that whether electrolytes are the villains is still a mystery to us.

The Genetic Approach

There is significant evidence that some forms of depression may be transmitted through a family's bloodline. This is important because it leads from chemotherapy into the even more arcane subject of genetic engineering.

In 1969 Dr. George Winokur, of the University of Iowa College of Medicine, conducted a fascinating study showing that manic-depressives might pass on either manic-depressive or depressive tendencies. Winokur speculated, on the basis of statistics, that the problem might reside in an arm of the X chromosome—the same arm that carries color blindness and a red blood cell antigen called Xga. What made Winokur's theory compelling at the time was that it seemed to explain a baffling phenomenon—namely, that women seem much more prone to depression, while men are more likely to become alcoholics.

That this is true has long been recognized. Depression has always been the scourge of women. Since ancient times, in psychiatric hospitals the depressive female has rated high on the admission list. For years we blamed this on cultural conditions, persecution or social ranking. Moreover, since men tended to gravitate toward alcohol, we thought that maybe we were dealing with a detection or labeling discrepancy.

There is still evidence that this may be true. Alcohol and depression may be related, with women being conditioned to seek help from the medical profession, while men, who "don't need help," simply crawl into a bottle somewhere.

What Winokur suggested was something deeper: He postulated a genetic origin behind female depression, and that alcoholism, which is also inheritable, might have a similar, but male-oriented, etiology. You see, X-chromosome traits are by nature "sexist." That is, a mother can pass them to either daughter or son, but a father can only pass them to his daughter, meaning more women will inherit the genes in the X factor. Theoretically, if X chromosomes are to blame for depression, we would have about twice as many female as male depressives. While that is a bit neat and oversimplified, the statistics show that it is not unreasonable.

Reporting recently in *Resident & Staff Physician,* Dr. Myrna M. Weissman, an epidemiologist at Yale, cited five different studies of sex ratios in depression giving women a lead of just about that proportion. The most even-handed ratio, out of Baltimore, Maryland, showed women leading men by 60 percent. A United States survey showed 238 depressed females for every 100 male depressives.

As I say, this theory is still highly inconclusive, because there are contradictory findings that keep muddying the water. We do, for example, find depressed father-son pairings, which would not be the case were X chromosomes the only factor. Furthermore, a subsequent study has pretty well ruled out Dr. Winokur's gene location. The gene was not found near the color-blindness gene or in the area of the Xga red-cell antigen.

But there is substantial evidence that depression *is* inheritable, whether or not we have located the gene. Many studies on sets of twins leave little or no doubt about the genetic indicators. We have found that among twins who have been reared apart, there is a 67 percent concordance in depressive disorders. We have also learned that when one twin is depressed, the other will seldom possess any mania traits.

Where does this leave us? From the standpoint of research it leaves us with many questions to answer. Obviously we have only scratched the surface. It will be years before our hypotheses can be proven definitely. From the standpoint of *treatment*, from the standpoint of helping people, we are light-years ahead of where we were twenty years ago. This means that if you are suffering from depression, you have an excellent chance for quick recovery.

6

More Depression

—The Manic Factor
—The Female Factor
—The Aging Factor

I feel as if I'm in a giant squirrel cage like they have at carnivals, where you are plastered to the side by centrifugal forces. If someone turned off the switch, I would fall to the bottom.
—Self-description by a manic-depressive

Mania is derived from the Greek word for madness, but, as in all psychiatric terminology, we have spent many years refining our semantics, slicing each aberration into ever-narrowing entities. Emil Kraepelin, the great nineteenth-century taxonomist, was the first to catalog manic-depression. He set it apart from schizophrenia, in which there were similar thought patterns but no depression syndrome. Kraepelin proposed that manic-depression was a cyclical adjunct of common depression. We now suspect that this is not the case. Manic-depression is a very distinct illness.

Recently psychiatrists honed the definition still further by calling manic-depression *bipolar depression*. This implies two opposing mood states and distinguishes it from regular depression, which is said to be *unipolar*.

In manic-depression there is an elevation of mood. Life becomes filled with wonderful potential. There are plans to be laid, dreams and schemes to be acted upon. Activity continues right into the sleeping hours. Insomnia develops. This, too, is okay. Who needs sleep when life is so wonderful? The victim feels nothing but joy and generosity—and, above all, the need to keep moving, to do things. Often the victim becomes more sex oriented. Promiscuity is likely to become part of the pattern. Nor is money an obstacle—he may squander his bank account on the most foolish enterprises. Family and friends may try to intercede, but their logic and reasoning seem irrelevant. The victim's speech gets disorganized; he becomes hostile and violent—in extreme cases he might even die of exhaustion.

People in the midst of a manic episode are hard to distinguish from other psychotics. They may be racing, disorganized, agitated, violent. They may have paranoid ideas. They may become hallucinatory. But the upswing always results in a horrifying freefall. Their schemes and ideas begin to unravel. They plummet from the heights of ecstasy to the darkest realms of despair and despondency.

For some reason age plays a role in this illness. The peak age for depression is forty to fifty, but in manic-depressives the age is lower, with the worst cases being in their twenties and thirties. Once again, women predominate. This may be due to a genetic factor. It has been clearly established that family history plays an important role in the incidence of mania.

Manic-depression seems to be more prevalent among endomorphs. These are people with round body shapes. Why this should be remains a mystery, but it may involve the endocrine system. We have also noticed that swings in mood seem to occur most frequently in fall and spring. It has been suggested by several authorities that this points to a link with ancient hibernation patterns.

103

Whatever the cause, manic-depression *is* controllable. Lithium is both a cure and a preventative. As such it is superior to all other psychotropics, including CPZ and the much-heralded antidepressants.

Lithium was discovered in 1817 by a scientist named Johan August Arfvedson while working in the laboratory of a Swedish chemist, Baron Jöns Jakob Berzelius. A silvery-white substance that appears as a salt, lithium is the lightest of earth's alkali metals. It is extremely hard and liberates exceptional energy when placed in water, to which it is attracted.

The distribution of lithium is almost universal. It appears in more than 150 minerals. It is found in seawater, in fresh water, in plant life—it is even found in tobacco and sunshine. The uses of lithium go far beyond psychiatry. As a power source it is almost unparalleled. Most modern pacemakers run on lithium, and NASA has found that it makes an excellent rocket fuel!

It may seem strange that such an unlikely substance could be of benefit to a manic-depressive, but it illustrates how the human race is but a very small part of an infinite ecosystem. The seas, the trees, the earth's crust itself are integral parts of our life on this planet. They not only contribute to our physical well-being but to the more ethereal concepts of mood and psychology. I said at the beginning that some of our ideas might be unsettling. We may not like to think of a metal as contributing to personality. Yet this common little alkali, more abundant than zinc, can send some people to the moon and alter other people's thought processes.

Lithium's effectiveness is about 80 percent, even taking possible spontaneous remissions into account. Its effectiveness stands up against the most rigorous challenges, including "double blind" and "double blind crossover" tests. The *way* in which it cures is still mysterious. Does it cure through electrolytes, transmitters or the endocrine system? It has an effect on all three of these processes, but which is the curative one remains an enigma to us.

There are other enigmas: In the early days of lithium, it was believed to work solely on the mania syndrome, not as an antidepressant but as an antipsychotic, perhaps analogous to Thorazine. We now know that this is not the case. Lithium does

104

help alleviate depression. While it flattens the mania in manic-depressives, it is not nearly so effective against schizophrenia.

You can see the quandary this puts us in. We are curing people through the theater of their symptoms. We guess at the mechanisms behind the curtain on the basis of the activities being presented along the footlights. The problem is that this can be misleading. Mania, apparently, has different mechanisms. The same behavior in two different sick people might have entirely different causes and origins. We know that lithium has an effect on electrolytes, that it may act as a substitute for potassium and sodium. We also know that it alters cortisol levels and seems to deplete certain relevant neurotransmitters. The end result is that if a doctor puts a manic-depressive on a program of lithium, the mania will subside, the depression will be elevated and the patient will function with a more even temperament.

Oddly, for some patients this is not a blessing. For them, mania is terrific—it is the thrill of their lives. They do not welcome the prospect that a drug will deprive them of that high, since, in the maelstrom of their existence, mania has become a positive. They would rather have a drug that eliminates the low spots and keeps them flying in a euphoric state. They are unable to see that this very euphoria creates much of the misery they experience.

When a psychiatrist treats a manic-depressive, he must first confirm his diagnosis. He will ask the patient about his feelings and mood changes. He will take his family's history and may ask for a medical checkup. Once it is determined that lithium is called for, he will put the patient on a therapeutic dosage. This is designed to raise the lithium in the blood to a level under what would be considered toxic.

The doctor monitors the blood levels regularly. The blood is analyzed with a flame photometer, an instrument that measures light. An expert can use it to determine lithium content.

Once a therapeutic level is established, the patient will notice a change in his mood. He should feel somewhat less hyper, more in control of his life. His depressed periods will probably seem somewhat less terrifying. Possibly he will also have some side effects. His speech might be slurred, his hands might tremble.

105

The latter can be controlled by administering a nerve blocker, but we would rather not do that, because the trembling is usually temporary.

Once a therapeutic level is established, the dosage will be dropped to a maintenance level. This level will also be periodically monitored and can be adjusted for effectiveness and comfort.

I mentioned earlier that lithium is toxic. This should not be of any great concern. There are a number of drugs—digitalis, for example—that are harmful in doses that exceed the therapeutic. Most side effects from lithium are innocuous and temporary. The patient may feel lethargic or nauseous or thirsty. This disappears after one or two weeks, and there is no reason to feel overly concerned about it. If the patient does take a lithium overdose and the blood level exceeds what is recommended, this can affect the central nervous system, causing a mild or moderate impairment of consciousness. The recommended treatment is to withhold lithium salt while increasing intake of sodium, or table salt. Sodium, you see, helps eliminate lithium, which is why patients on lithium must keep up their salt intake.

About the only time lithium may be contraindicated is among patients with heart trouble or a history of kidney ailment. It should also never be used as a salt substitute or among patients who have been put on a salt-free regimen.

The Female Depressions

The news that women have unique psychiatric problems may be viewed by some as a bit heretical. Am I implying that women are emotionally unstable? Am I saying that the male is psychically superior? Actually I'm not saying either of those things. I am saying that women and men are different. The organic differences, which are evident to everybody, lead naturally and inevitably to different psychiatric problems.

For many centuries doctors and feminists agreed that women's depressions were social in origin. They perceived the illness as either cultural or psychic, arising from feelings of inferiority. It's a comfortable notion that allows women to feel persecuted and men to indulge fantasies of superiority. Thinking that (a) women are being abused or (b) are not tough enough are simply two different ways of ignoring certain medical realities.

Since the switch in focus from the abstract to the physical, a new perception of women has begun to emerge. Their emotional problems are seen as real and well founded, but they can result from chemistry as well as other factors. This focus does not exclude or deny injustice, which can trigger or aggravate a depressed condition, but it says that there is probably a propensity for depression that can be explained through the female chemistry. In every period of history, in every culture, women have been twice as prone to mood disorders. This alone argues against social causes. One would expect to see a greater statistical variation.

Of course, the vast majority of women do not suffer from depression, have never had it and are never likely to. We are talking about a very small percentage, which happens to be twice the male percentage. So to use the depression factor as an argument against the Equal Rights Amendment or as an excuse to keep women suppressed in the job market would be about as specious as discriminating against men on the basis of the male propensity for heart attack.

There are three depressed states that are associated with women: postpartum, premenstrual and oral contraceptive. These are not separate illnesses; they are basically *one* illness that manifests itself in three separate circumstances. Postpartum depression strikes directly after childbirth. Premenstrual depression comes the week before menses. Oral-contraceptive depression is the most recent ailment, striking significant numbers who routinely take birth-control pills. Actually they are all endogenous depression. There is nothing pathologically different about them. They are the same illnesses men get, but with different mechanisms—and they are certainly not caused by psychological frailty.

POSTPARTUM DEPRESSION

In the Freudian days postpartum depression was considered purely psychological—arising from certain unconscious conflicts

107

that were psychodynamic and uniquely "female." In 1929 Dr. Gregory Zilboorg, a distinguished Freudian psychiatrist, conducted a study of postpartum depression that reflected his era's thinking. Childbirth was seen as a "loss of self." He described women who were depressed after childbirth as ambivalent and sadistic toward men. He accused them of having a castration complex and of having failed to resolve their oedipal complexes, views that were echoed by other psychiatrists. The woman was thought to feel inadequate as a mother and probably rejecting of her own mother as a positive role model.

There are undoubtedly cases in which Zilboorg's analysis of these conflicts is applicable. No one would deny that there are such women. But we have come to see postpartum depression as more biochemical, having all the earmarks of endogenous depression. The cause of this pathology is still a bit hazy, but I will describe what we currently think may give rise to depression in the maternity ward.

The organic changes during pregnancy and childbirth are dramatic and diffuse throughout the body. The ordeal of carrying and launching a new life causes severe alterations in the female biosystem. There are hormone changes. Estrogen and progesterone levels shoot up during pregnancy, then drop after childbirth. In addition other substances increase during pregnancy, such as *thyroxin*, which helps set the body's metabolic rate. Too much thryoxin leads to overactivity. A condition develops called hyperthyroidism. Too little thyroxin causes sluggishness and moodiness—an illness like depression, only with an accompanying weight gain.

Could it be that the changes in these important hormones are what throw a new mother off her equilibrium? The rise and fall of these important substances might send shock waves through the nerves and into the limbic system.

Another vital hormone is estrogen. One of the prime determinants of feminine behavior, it lowers one's proclivity toward hostility and violence. One thing we know through animal studies is that estrogen inhibits MAO. In other words, it has a kind of elevating effect not unlike Marplan, Nardil or Parnate. Could it be that during the hours and days following childbirth, when the estrogen level falls off by about 40 percent, the sudden return of MAO causes a transmitter depletion that sends the psyche into a tailspin? This has yet to be corroborated through proper studies, but it does indicate a promising path of research. It might mean that the most effective weapon for fighting this illness is not tricyclics but MAO inhibitors.

It will take several more years to find the answers to these questions. In the meantime here is a checklist of exactly what we do know. The new mother who is fearful or anxious may find comfort in some of these observations:

1. Postpartum depression is a temporary illness occurring in some 20 percent of recorded childbirths. It is nothing more than endogenous depression, with its roots, or etiology, tracing back to certain hormonal changes.
2. Most women after childbirth—even those with little depression—manifest certain temporary behavioral changes. These appear in psychological tests, showing an increase of anxiety, neuroses and volatility.
3. Of those who are depressed, a very high percentage will be women who have suffered previous episodes. These women seem to possess a predisposition that makes them susceptible to this particular malady.
4. Postpartum depression is curable. It often responds to antidepressants. Where these are barred, or when there is extreme morbidity, it is one of the most responsive illnesses to electroshock therapy.
5. The postpartum depressive is neither evil nor inadequate. It is her body, not her mind, that is playing tricks on her, and with proper treatment and a supportive family, within a few weeks or months she will probably be herself again.

To give you some idea of the mechanisms of this illness, let me borrow a case study from my own private practice. While the circumstances are unique to this particular case, they are fairly representative of the postpartum syndrome.

Several years ago a young woman came to me suffering from all the symptoms of endogenous depression. I prescribed a routine drug-therapy program with a supplemental treatment of psychoanalysis.

The young woman was a Catholic with a religious upbringing. As an adult she had met and married a Protestant. She quickly became pregnant, but since they did not want children yet, at the urging of her husband, she agreed to an abortion.

Shortly after the abortion, she became despondent. This is when she first appeared in my office. Analysis revealed a deep-seated anger aimed against her husband for "what he has done to me." In her mind, he had turned her against her parents. She held him responsible for the loss of her religion. She also believed that he had caused her to sin, performing an act that was troubling to her conscience.

In due course we confronted these problems, and soon her depression began to recede. Despite her anger she still loved her husband, and the affection between them provided a foundation to build upon.

Two years later, with those events in the past, the couple decided to have a baby. This time the pregnancy went full term and the woman had the baby that had previously been denied her. Only now, instead of feeling joy, the woman relapsed into a postpartum depression. All the old hostilities resurfaced, along with the same symptoms she had had when I first encountered her.

The lesson, of course, is reasonably obvious: It returns us to the connection between the mind and the body. This woman suffers from a *chemical* susceptibility that manifests itself through certain *psychological* symptoms. During normal times she loved her husband. He was supportive and affectionate and would have done nothing to harm her. Indeed, between the abortion and the childbirth, theirs had been a happy, healthy, compatible relationship. But when something happened to traumatize the woman— whether that trauma was abortion or the advent of motherhood— her body sent out chemical messages that were decoded into hostility against "the man who has done this to me." It would be foolish to deny the psychodynamics, to imply that her condition was solely chemical, but it would be equally foolish, considering our present knowledge, to say that resentment was at the root of everything. Obviously this woman requires two kinds of therapy: She requires *chemo*therapy to restore her chemistry, and she requires *psycho*therapy to give her tools to cope and to prevent further damage to her marital relationship.

The standard drug therapy for postpartum depression is the same as for endogenous depression, except in cases where the mother is breast-feeding, in which case additional care must be exercised. The usual drugs of choice are the same as for other depressions: tricyclics or MAO inhibitors. In addition, a doctor may prescribe *triiodothyronine*, which helps restore the levels of thyroxine. Only in severe cases, where suicide is feared or where for some reason the drugs don't seem to take hold, might the doctor recommend a series of shock treatments—which, as I hope I have made clear, is not grounds to become panic-stricken.

PREMENSTRUAL DEPRESSION

Although premenstrual depression, like postpartum depression, is another form of endogenous depression, there is no correlation between the two to hint that menstrual distress is an omen against childbirth. On the contrary, the two don't seem to be linked. Some postpartum depressives report menstrual irregularity, but there is no reason to assume that trouble during menses is a predictor that the woman will have problems following childbirth.

Since the dawn of medicine premenstrual depression has hit all kinds of women in all kinds of social climates. Studies in the United States and England show that about a third of young women suffer some form of premenstrual distress. About 10 percent of these suffer so acutely that their everyday activities are disturbed. And about 60 percent of women's violent acts in prison are committed by inmates during the week before menstruation.

By its very nature premenstrual distress points to problems in the pituitary and hypothalamus. These are the glands that regulate the clock mechanisms not only of menses but of other bodily functions. In addition, there is evidence that moodiness preceding menstruation is probably tied to hormone production. In this regard it is similar to postpartum depression and intimately linked to the endocrine system.

The ovulation cycle takes twenty-eight days, eight of which constitute the premenstrual and menstrual period. During these eight days a number of women experience recurring discomfort, including depressed feelings. During the twenty-eight-day cycle there are two peak estrogen periods: an *ovulation peak,* which occurs around midcycle, and the *luteal peak,* which occurs on or about day twenty-one. Estrogen, you'll recall, is an MAO inhibitor, which shuts off production of monoamine oxidase. As the estrogen level falls off, presumably MAO returns. This may destroy neurotransmitters, creating depression and mood changes.

But estrogen has other interesting functions. We know, for example, from carefully controlled studies that it lowers the seizure threshold in both rats and humans, making them more susceptible to convulsions and spasms. On the other hand, progesterone, another female hormone, *raises* one's defenses against seizure or convulsion. It seems to have a sedative effect, nature's equivalent of a general anesthesia.

Progesterone begins to be secreted at midcycle, reaching highest concentration on about day twenty-one. After that the level diminishes rapidly, at just about the same time estrogen diminishes. It is very possible that the rise of progesterone produces a feeling of mild sedation. When it drops, after about the third week of the cycle, it might create a discomfort not unlike drug withdrawal.

Estrogen production during the first fourteen days inhibits MAO and causes a rise in transmitter activity. It also creates feelings of pleasantness, activation and sexual arousal leading up to ovulation. During the third week of the cycle, progesterone takes over, although the body is still producing estrogen. The entire system becomes mildly sedated—so mildly that it is virtually indiscernible. At the end of the third week, both hormones diminish. The pleasantness is gone, and so is the sedation. This is when, often unbeknownst to the woman, she becomes irritable, anxious, depressed, even violence prone.

Since premenstrual depression is of short duration, it is not appropriate to take antidepressants, although, if anxiety accompanies the feeling of depression, a doctor might prescribe an anxiolytic. Perhaps the best thing a woman with this problem can do is simply note it and be aware of it. She may even want to get a calendar and keep a diary of her experiences during the days of her menstrual cycle. This might help anticipate mood swings. It might also help in personal relationships. By pinpointing the days that are likely to cause trouble, a woman might cope more effectively with situations that could create unhappiness. In some cases diuretics, stimulants or progesterone can be helpful.

Depression and Aging

If you were to look at out-of-date psychiatry texts, you would find vast sections on depression and aging. Concomitant with the suspicion that sex was linked to mood changes, there was also a feeling that time was a factor. Menopausal depression was considered a separate illness. It prevailed among women, but men also seemed affected by it. It was thought that beyond midlife there were unique biological changes that resulted in mood swings unknown in younger people.

The label for this phenomenon was *involutional melancholia,* meaning the depression that struck during physical and sexual atrophy. No one could deny that such behavioral changes existed, and we spent many years trying to find the causes for it.

More recently, however, since the advent of mood-changing drugs, we have brought more stringent empiricism to bear. We have concluded that the depression that attacks during menopause is virtually identical to endogenous depression. It has all the same symptoms, all the same complaints, all the same effects on appetite and sleep patterns—and, most important from the standpoint of the patient, it responds to similar chemotherapy.

Aging alone can be the source of unhappiness. It is a time of fear, of diminished or lost faculties. But these feelings alone do not constitute depression. And there is no drug on earth that can make you *un*disappointed. What *is* true, however, is that menopausal depression is often accompanied by unique psychological symptoms. This is particularly true in our culture, in which menopause can be acutely distressing.

When feelings of distress accompany *physical* depression—in other words, when they are associated with the vegetative symptoms—it is of course important to get relief on both fronts, through chemotherapy and traditional psychotherapy. Suicide statistics among women rise sharply in this period. For that matter, so do those for both drug abuse and overdose. A woman must be candid in talking with her doctor and follow instructions concerning drug therapy to the letter.

Among men this age period is not so easily defined. There is still a debate as to whether men undergo menopause. There are chemical changes that do take place, but their role in depression is extremely conjectural. Most male depressives have a history of the illness. It seems only to have returned during middle age. The one exception might be that relatively rare man who has predicated his identity on his potency and his sexual prowess. For him, of course, some sort of analysis seems called for. For others it is a much more routine sort of therapy. Most antidepressants work fine on these patients as long as there are no unusual, extenuating circumstances.

Beyond middle age, beyond the years of menopause, depression can also hit the retired and elderly. This is a very special subgroup, because both treatment and diagnosis can be so complicated.

I think it should be said on behalf of the elderly that their depression often rises from valid circumstances. Their faculties are impaired, they are often homeless, their friends may be dead, they are financially straitjacketed. Our society is not very humane toward the elderly. They are put through indignities that the young would find insufferable. Therefore, their depression is often reactive, arising naturally and inevitably from their bitter circumstances.

Beyond this, there are other problems. How do we know that an old person is depressed? How do we know that it's not senility or a dozen other illnesses that can mimic depression? In psychiatry

114

there is a term, *pseudodementia,* meaning a "false senility" often found among older people. Many older people have been interned for senility when, as it has subsequently been discovered, they are suffering from depression.

One way we now test for pseudodementia is to try the patient on an antidepressant. If that doesn't work, then he may have some organic illness that is altering his behavior. He may have Alzheimer's disease, a leading cause of senility, or kidney disease or some sort of heart problem. Or he may be reacting to medication, which is seldom tailored to the needs of enfeebled people.

However, many "senile" people are actually depressed. When you put them on tricyclics, they suddenly become "young" again. It was one of the sadder shortcomings of predrug psychiatry that there was no reliable way to differentiate these maladies.

Another problem almost unique among the elderly is vitamin deficiency and poor nutrition. Yes, these too contribute to our mental well-being, as will be explained in more detail in Chapter 10. You see, neurotransmitters have to come from somewhere. They are constructed from other substances that act as "precursors." The process is extremely detailed and complicated, like the construction of a house out of dissimilar building materials. Serotonin and norepinephrine, for example—two of our most important transmitters, whose roles are highly suspect in the etiology of depression—are derived from two nutrients found in proteins: tryptophan and tyrosine.

The substances that cause these transformations to take place—that act, if you will, as the body's construction crew—are the numerous enzymes found in every cell and, at least in some cases, in the food on our dinner tables. Our knowledge of the construction is still somewhat hazy—there are innumerable contributors to each metamorphosis—but we can isolate at least two "weak links" that seem to afflict the elderly much more than younger people.

One weak link is vitamin B_{12}. Another is a substance called folic acid. A deficiency in one or both of these agents appears in about 10 percent of elderly depressives. The problem, we believe, is in the diet. Many elderly people tend to buy cheap foods that are easy to prepare. Some will also fill up on sweets and candies, having lost their ability to enjoy more nutritious items.

Admittedly, this might be part of a vicious cycle, in that depressed people also tend to have poor appetites—their taste buds are "flattened" and they are often too lethargic to take the time to cook properly. But deficiencies in B_{12} and folic acid have been noted most commonly among elderly people. Supplementing their diet with one or both of these substances is often quite effective in relieving their depression.

Another possible contributor to depression among the aged is a marked upswing in MAO. This is the enzyme that destroys neurotransmitters and that itself is the target of MAO inhibitors. Why elderly patients have more MAO is still a matter of scientific conjecture, but we suspect there may be some other deficiency that affects the ability to regulate MAO activity.

Whatever the causes of depression among the aged, the treatment of their illness requires a unique set of guidelines. Old people cannot take the same kind of medicine that is administered so freely to vigorous young people. As you will recall from our discussion in earlier chapters, all these drugs have a variety of side effects. They work throughout the autonomic nervous system to create problems in everything from blood pressure to bowel movement. In a young or middle-aged person, these may be minor nuisances, but to an elderly patient the effects can be disastrous. Therefore, we will often give older patients lower dosages and monitor their reactions more frequently.

Not only can drugs be overpowering for old people, they can also result in paradoxical reactions. What this means is that the drug's true effect may be the very opposite of what the doctor intended. One of the best examples of this is Valium. In he population at large Valium works as a tranquilizer, but among many people age sixty-five and over, Valium sometimes works as a stimulant—and alarmingly so. I have seen elderly patients react violently to Valium. They become wound up, agitated, incoherent. One would have thought that instead of being given a calming agent they were in the psychotic stages of a bad LSD trip.

In cases of very severe depression in which for some reason

drugs may be considered unwise, ECT can be used for an elderly patient, as long as there are no ailments to contraindicate it. Of course ECT for the aged has other ramifications. Will the family be willing to go along with it? For that matter, does the patient herself have the will to live beyond her present predicament?

At present our society seems to wish to defer the problem of the aged. With regret we put our parents in nursing homes and grit our teeth until the "ordeal" is over. But how long this can continue is problematical. The exposés crowd in around us—stories of neglect and abuse by staff members, of oversedation in the name of orderliness. As the "baby boom" products who are now in their thirties move through our society like a lump through a python, they will soon be confronting the decline of their own powers and may have grave trepidations about the fate that awaits them. Perhaps then we will pay more attention to the elderly. Perhaps then we will refocus the priorities of our medical care. It is a problem the surface of which we have only begun to scratch. I hope that in the future we will pay more attention to it.

7

The Question-Mark Illnesses—Anxiety, Panic, Phobias and Compulsions

Until now this narrative has been marked by optimism. We have revealed some discoveries that have reshaped medicine, we have discussed some conditions that were formerly baffling but, through the genius of science, are now less mysterious to us. As was foretold at the beginning, it has been a journey of promise. Despite a few murky edges, it has followed a logical pattern. But now I'm about to confuse the issue by showing how everything we've learned is but a flicker in the darkness.

Anxiety and Panic

In the discussion of affective disorders, I said that drugs seem to work on certain neurotransmitters, that as you increase their activity your mood goes up and as you decrease their activity you slump into lethargy. On the high end of the scale are hyperactivity and mania. On the low end are depression and sedation. The theory is very simple and logical and would seem to provide a blueprint for other disorders.

The trouble is that the theory doesn't transfer. What works on one illness doesn't work on another. In fact, identical therapies don't even work on identical symptoms when those symptoms are connected to other behavioral modes!

Take anxiety, for example—a common enough illness and one whose subjective effects are universally recognized. Anxiety is fear, tension, foreboding, the eerie dread of what the unknown has in store. In psychiatry we distinguish anxiety from fear by the appropriateness and specificity of the object of the emotion. To be afraid of *something* is human and constructive. To be anxious about *nothing* is debilitating and nerve-racking.

Of course few will admit that they are anxious about nothing. If questioned, they will create a target for their fear. They are afraid of death. They are afraid of being alone. They are afraid of being done in by some indescribable happenstance. There is nothing wrong with feeling anxious over some things. Who wouldn't feel anxious in the face of major surgery? Whose heartbeat might not race a little faster while sitting in a plane that's about to leave the runway? What drives a person to the psychiatrist's office is experiencing the same feelings at home in the living room—when the most innocuous and familiar scenes and events make a person's palms get sweaty and his knees buckle under him.

If anxiety—or for that matter any mood that makes your heart leap—is assumed to be an aspect of the "fight-or-flight" phenomenon, we might logically suppose that it is akin to mania, an internalized analog of hyperactivity. If that were true we might treat it with lithium. Or we might permanently control it with some sort of sedative. The last thing in the world that would logically cure it is an antidepressant, which we assume to be a mood elevator.

But, ironically, such is not the case. *There is no drug cure for chronic anxiety.* On the other hand, there are certain panic disorders that mysteriously respond to antidepressants.

The following is a classical animal experiment, a refinement of the old Pavlovian technique that is used to illustrate the enigma of anxiety. The experiment is a perfect example of the mystery that confronts us.

A dog is trained, upon hearing a bell, to jump from a grid to avoid a shock. After a brief training period the shocks are discontinued, but when the dog hears the bell, he continues to jump. Over a period of time this behavior becomes automated. The dog's movements become increasingly graceful. He has learned to respond to the anticipation of pain, but his response is no longer aroused or frightened.

This behavior resembles neurotic behavior. The dog is mechanically performing a ritual. *Only when the researcher prevents him from jumping does the dog begin to show signs of anxiety.*

If we were to assume that an "unconscious anxiety" exists which only becomes manifest at the blocking of a ritual, we could deduce that an antianxiety drug might lower this feeling and eliminate the ritual. In reality this is not the case. Taking a Valium or Librium would not induce the conditioned dog to change his behavior. The drug would only reduce his trembling and quaking.

This is why the minor tranquilizers are *not* the panacea some people think they are. They do not keep a person from being neurotic, they only dampen and ameliorate some of the more obvious physical symptoms. The only sound way to eliminate the anxiety itself is to change the behavior through psychotherapy, which in turn has its roots in traditional analysis.

It may seem ironic in view of the present lexicon in which *anxiety* has become almost cocktail-party chic, that it was not always considered an emotional ailment but was for years assumed to be physiological. During the Civil War it was noted that soldiers were suffering strange symptoms. Their hearts malfunctioned. They complained of chest pains. They had diarrhea, palpitations and other infirmities. Mystified, the doctors conjectured that it was a newfangled nerve ailment. They gave it the label "soldier's heart" and presumed that it was caused by exertion and battle fatigue.

With the advent of Freud's theories the surgical concept gave way to speculation that the disorder was emotional. Freud proposed that "soldier's heart" was the result of fear—an aversion to having one's head blown off. The fear was complicated by societal strictures. A man could not confess to being a coward. He

120

must continue to march, he must continue to fight—but inside he was being physically lacerated.

Freud arrived at his conclusions through a theory of analysis that gave birth to such concepts as *libido* and *repression*. Much of anxiety he saw as sexual in origin, often tracing it back to the earliest developmental stages. There are certain wishes, he proposed, of a sexual or destructive nature, that for one reason or another must not be acted upon. These we repress through the use of the *superego*, which is the conscience we have developed through our roles as social animals. Often such repression takes a terrible toll on us. The id and the libido cry out for recognition. We experience urges of destruction and/or sex that can sometimes be converted into maladaptive behavior rituals.

Anxiety as we know it falls into four major categories. The first is *superego anxiety*, which is analogous to "conscience," or the guilt we suffer from misdeeds or wrongdoing. *Castration anxiety* is a fear of bodily mutilation. Obviously it is rooted in sexual confusion. In men it frequently involves homosexuality. The third type is *separation anxiety*, fear of loss of an important relationship. The fourth major category is *impulse anxiety*, which is fear of our destructive impulses.

Ancillary to these four major categories are a host of other anxiety conditions, many of which have obvious causes, such as losing one's job or going to a dentist's office. Sometimes anxiety turns into *panic*, a sudden, exacerbated distress. A person will suffer dizziness or a choking feeling and feel the need to rush to a window to keep from smothering. (When fear or anxiety focuses on one situation—such as height or crowds or stray dogs or insects—the victim suffers from a *phobia*. In the view of psychiatrists, phobia is a separate phenomenon.)

To return to anxiety and panic, a discussion of the enigmas we're faced with is in order.

If antipsychotics like CPZ have unpleasant effects on nonpsychotics, then presumably they wouldn't help the "normal" person who is only suffering from some form of anxiety.

121

But they do, sometimes.

If a "normal" person, suffering from anxiety, appears tense, distressed and unusually agitated, then presumably giving her an antidepressant would only serve to exacerbate whatever is troubling her.
But it doesn't, sometimes.

If you have an acutely ill schizophrenic patient, where the first drug of choice is a major tranquilizer, it makes no sense at all to use an antidepressant, because that will only make him more hyper and elevated.
But it doesn't, sometimes.

If a nonpsychotic is suffering from panic—say, agoraphobia, the fear of crowds—it should be relieved by giving him the very same drug (CPZ) that relieves panic in a person suffering hallucinations.
But it isn't, ever.

When a doctor treats anxiety, a prescription for pills will be no more than a palliative. The pills will calm the jitters, they will relax the muscles, but they will have no effect on the source of the discomfiture. To cure anxiety one needs nondrug therapy. It might be analysis or some other type of treatment, but the patient must identify his neurotic rituals and establish new patterns that will help avoid conflict.

If the symptoms are acute and the patient cannot function, the doctor may prescribe a relaxant like Valium. But this should only be done on a short-term basis, to help ease the patient into a program of therapy. In July of 1980, a government edict advised all MDs to limit the period that patients are on Valium because of the increasing evidence of addiction and dependency. This edict was not binding, it was only advisory, but the majority of physicians will undoubtedly follow it. Only if there are extraordinary circumstances should a doctor renew any patient's Valium prescription.

Illnesses in Which Anxiety Plays a Role

reactive anxiety (in which the cause of anxiety is known)
anxiety neurosis (in which the cause of anxiety may not
   be known)
phobia with spontaneous anxiety attacks
phobia associated with specific objects or situations
obsessive-compulsive neurosis
depersonalization neurosis (feelings of unreality)
hypochondriasis
anxious depression
schizophrenia

Another drug sometimes used for anxiety is *propranolol*, a nerve-blocking agent. Propranolol's trade name is Inderal, and it is sometimes given to patients on lithium. Propranolol is a *beta blocker*. It blocks one type of postsynaptic receptor, called the beta receptor, in the sympathetic nervous system.

Propranolol is a major breakthrough in medicine, particularly for cardiac and blood-pressure patients. It is an alternative to drugs such as quinidine, which was the former drug of choice for people with arrhythmia. Before propranolol about all you could do for an angina patient was give him a drug that dilated his blood vessels. This, of course, would lower his blood pressure, but it had other effects not nearly so salutory. Propranolol works on the sympathetic nervous system, which is the system associated with exercise and stress. It has a calming effect on the heart during exertion but little effect during inactivity.

Until now propranolol's use in psychiatry has been of secondary, perhaps even tertiary, importance. Trade ads for Inderal and other beta blockers cannot mention their effects on anxiety. This is soon to change. Propranolol looks excellent for the treatment of anxiety—or, more precisely, the *physical* symptoms of anxiety, such as palpitations, cold sweats and chest constriction.

A word here about my attitude toward a treatment such as this, which has yet to be approved by the FDA: a doctor does not have to await such approval, as long as she can cite valid scientific evidence. The practice of modern medicine has become extremely complicated. It is developing so rapidly that one can hardly keep up with it. Particularly this is true of pharmacology, where there are literally thousands of drugs from which a doctor can choose. The average doctor judiciously shies away from drugs with which she is not familiar. She may have read about them, she may know them in theory, but she will be leery about using them until they have an established track record. The FDA is akin to a clearinghouse. It works as a pipeline between researchers and practitioners. It tells the doctor whether there is now sufficient evidence to use a certain drug with reasonable impunity.

The average doctor with a busy practice relies on this agency to make such judgments. To go off on her own, without the approval of the profession, would be extremely dangerous and leave the doctor open to lawsuit. But there are doctors like me whose job *is* research. We are associated with universities and research hospitals. We make it a point to try the most promising new substances in the hope that what we learn will serve as a model for other doctors.

So it is today with a drug like propranolol. Its use for anxiety is still in the test stage. But there is mounting evidence that it is both safe and effective, and my own experience lends support to this hypothesis.

Propranolol works on the peripheral nervous system. That is, it does not depress the central nervous system. In this it is unlike other tranquilizers, which cause sedation and a slowdown of the respiratory system. Propranolol is not for *all* anxious patients— only those with very acute physical symptoms and particularly those (à la the James-Lange theory, discussed on p. 59) whose symptoms themselves may be creating more anxiety. Stagefright is a perfect example of this. The symptoms (e.g., trembling) are what create the anxiety. Today, many actors and musicians who suffer from this handicap are being psychopharmacologically treated with doses of propranolol.

The Phobias

A classic phobia neurosis was reported many years ago by Pierre Janet, a contemporary of Sigmund Freud. Janet wrote about a 25-year-old man who was crossing the Place de la Concorde in Paris one day when he felt a strange sensation of dread. His breathing became rapid and he felt as if he were suffocating; his heart was beating violently and his legs were limp as if half-paralyzed.

From the time of that first episode on, he took a great dislike to the Place de la Concorde and decided he would not risk going there again alone. However, a short while after the same sensation of anxiety recurred on the Invalides Bridge, and then in a street.

Eventually he was not able to cross any square. Whenever he came to a square, he would begin to tremble and breathe heavily, develop tics and repeat the absurd phrase: "Mama, Rata, bibi, bitaquo, I'm going to die." His wife had to hold him tightly by the arm, and then he would calm down and cross the square without further incident. In the end, his wife had to accompany him everywhere, even when he went to the toilet.

Today we call this *agoraphobia*, and it is one of the most debilitating of all neuroses. Literally speaking, it means "fear of the marketplace," and the people who suffer from it number in the millions.

As established before, phobias are *not* anxiety. They are triggered by one certain object or circumstance. Sometimes they are accompanied by spontaneous panic attacks, and often they become part of a person's avoidance system. Anxiety may eventually become part of the picture, of course, because a person will become afraid of having a recurrence of panic. But we have learned from our attempts to treat such people with drugs that panic and anxiety are quite dissimilar entities.

Some of the most familiar questions quiz-show emcees ask involve the arcane labels we have given to phobias. Actually, these go back to the old taxonomists, who had a compulsive desire to put labels on everything. There is *erythrophobia*, which is the fear of blushing. Fear of being buried alive is *taphophobia. Ailurophobia* is the fear of cats, and *belonophobia* means that you can't stand needles. If you survive all these, you might become *siderodromophobic*, which means that you are absolutely panicked at the thought of a railroad train, or, if you are unusually exotic, you might be *triskaidekaphobic*, which means that you are terrified of having thirteen at your dinner table.

The list of such phobias goes on and on. There is virtually nothing that one can't be afraid of. And if you are one of those unfortunates who is afraid of everything, there's a name for that, too—*pantaphobia*.

The list of types of anxieties on page 123 illustrates that there are different anxieties attached to different phobias. Some of them are obviously sexual in nature; others are associated with annihilation. In the case of a person having agoraphobia, this seems to be connected with separation anxiety. Although the majority of agoraphobics are women, a larger percentage of phobics in general are male.

There is a path that phobias seem to take, as is illustrated in Pierre Janet's example. Typically, a phobia begins with a specific incident and spreads out in widening circles of fearfulness. At an early age a person may become afraid of something—let's assume it's something common, like height. He is on the roof of a building or at the end of a diving board, and suddenly he is gripped with a feeling of terror. His first reaction may be to avoid that locale again. He will stay off rooftops or the ends of high diving boards. But soon it may encompass all things that are elevated—stepladders, roller coasters, the top floors of office buildings.

One way that phobias differ from anxiety is that *the victim is totally conscious of his fear*. He knows *what* he fears (although he may not know *why* he fears it), and he understands perfectly the irrational nature of it. That is why it does absolutely no good to try to reason with a phobic person. He knows quite well how illogical he is being, but he is totally at a loss as to what to do about it.

Many phobias are not very serious. The majority of phobics never see a psychiatrist. If they are afraid of airplanes, they simply take trains. If they are claustrophobic, they avoid crowded elevators. But there are some phobias that can be absolutely devastating. Agoraphobia is one example. Another phobia that can

126

be seriously debilitating is the fear of eating, or *anorexia nervosa*.

In his bestseller *Tinsel*, novelist William Goldman describes a character named Ginger, who is anorexic. She is so horrified by the idea of food that, even when she does eat, she quickly regurgitates it. Anorexia nervosa is something more than a phobia, but it is often accompanied by phobic attitudes. It appears in young women, usually teenagers, and is sufficiently serious that some patients die from it.

Another constricting phobia, *mysophobia*, might be called the Howard Hughes phobia—the fear of germs. The patient becomes so obsessive about dirt that she sees a threat to life in literally everything around her. Because a phobia like this can be all-pervasive, it may appear similar to free-floating anxiety—except that in the case of the phobic there is a specific enemy, even though that enemy is invisible and ubiquitous.

If you set out to construct a theory about phobia, you might come up with the ivory-tower conclusion that it is an extreme manifestation of anxiety neurosis, only attached to a particular situation. The trouble is that this doesn't hold. About the only similarity is the incidence of panic. The treatment for one is not the same as for the other, and in both cases drugs are of limited value.

If you consider the element of panic alone, this is best combatted by antidepressants. Both MAO inhibitors and tricyclics like imipramine have been used effectively to alleviate panic attacks. Why this is we are not really sure. It undoubtedly involves certain neurotransmitters, but one of the ironies of the present state of the art is that drugs that lift your spirits can also prevent panic attacks.

Conversely, tranquilizers like Valium and Miltown—or for that matter alcohol and old-fashioned barbiturates—can be useful in lowering the symptoms of anxiety but are absolutely worthless in alleviating panic attacks. The problem with these kinds of drugs is that, in anticipation of the next panic attack, the victim may increase the dosage to relieve anxiety. As a result, there is a tendency for the victim to become addicted.

Perhaps someday an effective drug for treating phobias will be

127

developed, but until then we must resort to MAO inhibitors, tricyclics and nondrug therapy. At present the best technique available is a non-Freudian approach called *behavior modification*.

Behavior modification is based on the "learning theory," which has an honorable tradition dating back to Pavlov, the Russian scientist who pioneered the study of animal responses. Pavlov discovered that a dog's salivation, activated in response to the offering of food, could also be activated when no food was present by the ringing of a bell that had signaled previous feedings. Since then there have been other pioneers in learning theory—men like Wolpe, Skinner, Spence and Watson—and from their work has emerged a psychological subscience based upon the concept of *reinforcement*.

There are basically two ways of modifying behavior: You can reward a person for doing something right, or you can punish or hurt a person for committing a misdeed. It is possible that phobias are a kind of self-punishment—not purposeful, perhaps, but strong and effective—for the death of a loved one, the breaking of a sex taboo, even something more subtle but unpleasantly symbolic. If the event is accompanied by some neutral *stimulus*— say, the ringing of a church bell during one's mother's funeral—it is conceivable that the person could develop a phobia toward the ringing of church bells on other occasions.

In one of the most remarkable experiments in the history of psychology, a famous behaviorist named John B. Watson actually succeeded in creating a phobia in a happy, normal, well-adjusted infant. I won't defend the ethics of his experiment—they are bizarre at best and perhaps downright horrifying—but he actually did this back in 1920, and it sheds a fascinating light on behavior modification.

What Watson did was take an eleven-month-old child—a happy little boy by the name of Albert—and expose him to a number of "neutral" stimuli such as rats, rabbits, hats and Halloween masks. Albert responded agreeably to all of them. He saw no reason to be afraid of them. He laughed and cooed and reached out to touch them, showing not the least alarm or concern for his safety.

Then Watson introduced a rather fiendish element. He placed

an iron bar behind Albert's head. For the next few days, whenever a rat appeared, he struck the iron bar, making a fearful, clanging noise.

Albert's reaction was what one might expect. After a few such occurrences he began withdrawing from rats. The other objects caused him no alarm, but when a rat appeared, he trembled in terror of it.

Thus was planted the seed of a phobia. The very sight of a rat threw Albert into panic. Even when Watson stopped clanging the bar, if a rat appeared, Albert scrambled to avoid it.

So far this may not seem very earthshaking, but what happened next was profoundly illuminating. For within a very short time, with no further prompting, Albert's phobia spread to include all things with fur on them. When a rabbit appeared, he began to tremble. Even dogs, which he had liked, made him fearful and wary. By the end of the experiment, he was so upset that he could not stand to look at a bearded Santa Claus–face.

Behavior therapy, as it's practiced today, is usually an amalgam of various procedures. There's a new jargon to describe these procedures, but there is nothing very technical about the theories behind them. One procedure is called *desensitization*. In this various stimuli are graded in a hierarchy. The patient becomes "desensitized" to the least frightening stimulus and works his way up to that which most terrifies him.

Another technique is *reciprocal inhibition*. This pairs a phobia with a counteractive effect—something sufficiently calming, like muscle relaxation, to counterbalance the tension created by the stimulus.

Flooding is a technique in which the patient is required, usually in the presence of a supportive therapist, to face whatever is troubling her full-blast for periods extending up to several hours. *Implosion* is somewhat similar to flooding, only in this case the patient only imagines the fear stimulus. He fantasizes himself as being on an airplane or facing the rush hour on the New York City subway system.

The role of drugs is stopgap at best. They might relax a patient in preparation for therapy, or they might calm her physically to a sufficient degree that she is more pliable and willing to accept flooding or implosion. Often the doctor will prescribe a tranquilizer, but I caution again that this is only a Band-Aid. The patient must learn to let go of the prescription bottle and come to terms with the cause of the phobia.

Obsessive-Compulsive Neurosis

There are two other disorders that are somewhat akin to phobia but that manifest themselves in strangely opposite ways: One is a phenomenon we call *counterphobia,* and the other is *obsessive-compulsive neurosis.*

Counterphobics are familiar to everyone. These are people who have the same fears as phobics, but who, in their desire to conquer their terror, are irresistibly attracted to that which frightens them. Mountain climbers may be counterphobic. So may skydivers and other daredevils. Rather than remaining passive victims, they become active agents in the flouting of destruction. Children's games may be counterphobic. Have you ever watched a child play "doctor" with a doll? When she gives the doll an imaginary shot, she is countering her own fears by becoming the aggressor.

This is generally not a very serious disorder, in that it is rarely disruptive or frustrating to the sufferer. And even if it were, there is no drug that can prevent it, so the best that can be offered is supportive psychotherapy.

The other phenomenon is *obsessive-compulsive neurosis.* Obsession refers to an idea or a notion. It may be death, it may be a sex act, it may be anything that is viewed with abhorrence. It is not uncommon for the victim of this illness to have a fixed idea about the death of a loved one. It may be one's mother, one's father, one's children, but there is a vivid image of some horror that awaits.

To counteract this intolerable fate, the patient develops a ritualist compulsion. It is absurd, of course, and the patient knows this, but it nevertheless takes on a magical meaning. You may remember the childhood incantation, "Step on a crack, break your mother's back." This rhyme reflects how an obsessed person's mind works—the avoidance of cracks becomes all-consuming.

Obsessive-compulsive neurosis can be very serious. It can also be very interesting and sometimes bizarre. It is one of the favorite disorders of novelists and playwrights and has a long-standing tradition in Christian literature. Comic Flip Wilson created a character named Geraldine, who always used to say, "The devil made me do it!" In ages past many people said this and were thanked for their candor by being burned as witches.

A dramatic case of obsessive-compulsive neurosis concerns a man who worked on a factory assembly line and who developed a ritual: before he could solder one piece to another, he had to tap the workbench three times with his left hand and three times with his right, followed by stamping three times on the floor first with his left foot, then with his right. For a time this merely slowed his work performance. Gradually, however, an element of doubt crept into his mind. After completing a sequence of tapping and stamping, he would wonder: "Did I do it right? Am I sure I tapped three times?" He began to repeat the ritual to make sure it was perfectly done; but, the more he performed it, the greater his doubt. Before long, almost his entire working day was taken up by his rituals, and he was forced to leave his job.

There is something sadly ironic about stories like these. They are a cross between Dickens and the darkest of Kafka. But there is nothing comical in the misery of these people and the pain they feel in the web they have spun for themselves.

Obsessions and compulsions are akin to phobias—so much so that in his earliest formulations Freud mistakenly lumped them into the same general category, failing to see much distinction between them. And indeed in some ways they are rather similar. Both are psychic, without physical symptoms. Both revolve around an *idée fixe* and are often accompanied by shame and guilt feelings. But in other ways they are not alike. Obsessions, for example, do not create panic. And the treatments that we are even at this stage developing promise to be quite unlike those we are using for phobias.

131

All of us are compulsive to a minor degree. We all have rituals, which we refer to as habits, and when something prevents us from completing those rituals we may react with minor annoyance. Do you have a favorite side of the bed to sleep on? Do you knock on wood to ward off evil? Have you ever gone back to recheck a light switch even though you know very well you have already doused it? Then you have a dim awareness of obsessive-compulsiveness, and when it's highly magnified it becomes a disease. To break the ritual is almost impossible; it's as if you were telling the person not to breathe anymore.

Obsessions, like phobias, tend to begin early. Often we see them developing in children. A child becomes afraid of some impending disaster and, lacking the means to prevent it, develops a magical defense against it. By the time he grows up he may have hardened his behavior, particularly if his "magic" seems to have been effective, and by the time he comes into the psychiatrist's office, he may have developed a profile as unyielding as granite.

Obsessive people are fastidious. Often they are viewed as pillars of society. They are very neat, very logical, and their conversation may verge on pedanticism. Indeed, they are often intelligent people. Their average IQ is well above normal. They will sit in a chair, very prim and proper, and tell the doctor their problems as if reading from a textbook. They also tend not to be very emotional people. They like to feel they have everything in control. A place for everything and everything in its place is often one of their favorite catchphrases.

There is nothing "wrong" with this kind of person, who can be very productive and an excellent co-worker. I doubt if there is an office or successful business that has not benefited from an obsessive personality. But when the compulsions begin to take over—when elaborate rituals begin to drive out reality—such a valuable person may then become viewed as a liability.

Like phobics, obsessive-compulsives often have insight. They know very well the absurdity of their actions, and this usually causes them pain and embarrassment. Also, their profiles indicate that obsessive-compulsives often have loved ones who feel very close to them. Indeed, it is the loved ones who may suffer most, and this only increases the patients' embarrassment.

132

What can be done to help such people? It would be nice if we could give them a pill or an injection, something that would erase the idea that is upsetting them so that their defensive rituals would just fall by the wayside. Unfortunately such a pill has not yet been invented. The antipsychotic drugs don't seem to work, and while we can give patients Librium or Valium, these won't change their essential thought patterns. This leaves us with two other modes of treatment. One, of course, is behavior therapy. We have had some success using learning theory to "reteach" compulsives, just as we have our phobic patients.

But there is another kind of treatment that has been used successfully—but only in severe and crippling cases. It is a surgical procedure we call *leukotomy*. It is known more familiarly as *prefrontal lobotomy*.

Of all the words in the psychiatrist's dictionary, few are capable of arousing such emotionalism as *prefrontal lobotomy*. The thought of altering the brain may alarm even the most hardened practitioner. Psychosurgery (for that is what it is called) falls into the same troubled category as ECT: They are both referred to as somatic therapies, meaning that they are physical treatments of psychiatric disorders.

Psychosurgery is extremely unpopular and is seldom performed in the United States. Even should a patient desire it, there are laws and restrictions that curtail its practice. However, this is not true of all Western nations. Doctors in England, for example, view the procedure more leniently. I myself am extremely leery of it, but I believe it deserves more professional discussion.

Somatic surgery in modern medicine has a number of antecedents, one of which was the introduction of "malaria therapy" at about the turn of the century. This therapy was devised by an Austrian named Wagner von Jaurregg as a means of combatting the effects of syphilis. At the time about half of all patients in mental hospitals were suffering from psychosis as a result of venereal disease. Von Jaurregg made the astute observation that when a syphilitic came down with malaria, the aftereffect, during convalescence, was a marked reduction of the psychotic behavior associated with syphilis. What if malaria was an antidote for syphilis, or at least the paralysis and emotionalism that accom-

133

panied it? He decided to test this radical hypothesis by inducing malaria in a number of syphilitic mental patients.

Von Jaurregg took blood from patients who were suffering from malaria and injected it into syphilitics, treating them afterward with doses of quinine. The results of these tests were very promising. Indeed, the syphilitics *did* get better, and we now know that this was because of their fever; the extremely high temperature induced by malaria immobilized the bacteria that had been ravaging their brain cells.

The subsequent discoveries of sulfa and penicillin obviated the use of malaria therapy, but it was an early instance of biological treatment being brought to bear on a mental disorder.

Then in 1933 Egas Moniz of Portugal came up with an idea that would win him a Nobel Prize: He reasoned that the removal of frontal lobes in monkeys might reduce their aggressiveness without altering their intellect. The implications were obvious. What a boon to psychiatry! All you had to do was remove patients' frontal lobes. In 1936 Moniz performed the procedure, with initial results that looked extremely promising.

Enter Walter Freeman and James W. Watts, the former a neurologist from Washington, D.C., the latter a neurosurgeon who worked as his associate. In 1942 they began to perform lobotomies in the US. They experimented on many different areas of the brain. They also improved and streamlined the procedure until finally it became as routine as a haircut or an ear piercing.

Basically this is how it worked: The doctors jolted the patient with three bursts of electricity. Then they took two surgical "ice picks" and inserted them up through the patient's eye sockets. When the ice picks were approximately two inches deep, they maneuvered them about in a twirling manner, disconnecting the fine neural fibers between the frontal lobes and the area called the thalamus. The whole operation was very quick—Freeman could do it in about ten minutes—and this aspect was tremendously attractive to mental hospitals, which were overcrowded and had very few resources.

Between 1936 and the late 1950s, there were about fifty thousand lobotomies performed in this country. Freeman himself was involved in about four thousand of them, and some were performed by men who weren't even surgeons. Finally the authorities began to get alarmed. There were reports of bunglings, suicides, "zombies." There was a serious question of patients' rights and whether the victims had understood what was being done to them.

In the end it was not the moralists who put a stop to lobotomies but the dramatic discovery of chlorpromazine. Also, the idea of taking a pill was a lot less gruesome than sticking knives into eye sockets.

In 1977 the Department of Health, Education and Welfare (HEW) commissioned a study of psychosurgery, possibly in response to some journal editorials calling for a reexamination of this troubling field. There have been reports of late that psychosurgery shows promise—particularly in treating obsessive-compulsives. The operation has been greatly improved, but it still involves a small destruction of brain tissue.

I feel terribly ambivalent about this. I do not like the idea of damaging the brain. At best psychosurgery is a measure of our ignorance; at worst it is an echo of the horrors of naziism. Yet I must confess that on a few occasions I have been confronted with patients who were beyond medical therapy. Some of these patients have been obsessive-compulsives, so bound by ritual that their lives have become meaningless. Are we to let them rot? Drive them to suicide? Or should we partially relieve them, at the cost of impairment? I must confess I don't have the answer, and neither, I suspect, do most of my colleagues.

Clearly what is needed is a blue ribbon panel, probably associated with a university, to study the issue of psychosurgery and come up with guidelines concerning its use that will make sense to society. Right now, according to HEW, there is no consensus on its benefits and drawbacks, even among those surgeons who practice it. Different surgeons use different techniques, and they don't even agree on the patients who benefit from it. Aside from that, there are social questions. Who is to decide the candidacy of a patient? Who is to determine the amount of suffering that qualifies a person to lose a part of his or her brain functioning? It is similar to the decision a surgeon faces when he decides a woman must have a mastectomy, only in that case the issue has been relatively simplified by the clear and present danger to the patient's survival. Maiming a patient is always regrettable. These basic questions demonstrate how little we really understand about psychosurgery and how important it is that we learn more about it.

8

Schizophrenia—A Fine Madness?

Schizophrenia, as we have come to know it, was described as early as 1400 B.C. The Hindus believed that it was brought on by devils, and they left quite clear notes on the most prominent symptoms of it. Yet, ironically, it has remained a confusing illness. It has been called the psychiatric equivalent of cancer. It has been estimated that among Americans living today 1 in 100 will at some point be hospitalized for it.

A simple definition of schizophrenia is that it is a disorder of the brain causing a disturbance in logic, with an accompanying syndrome of abnormal behavior and an absence or inappropriateness of mood reaction. That's the way it reads in a textbook, but diagnosing it is something else. A schizophrenic may seem to be very similar to other types of sick people.

Our modern concepts of schizophrenia owe much to the efforts of Emil Kraepelin, a nineteenth-century German psychiatrist who distinguished the various symptoms and lumped them together in a coherent entity. This was not easy. There are many conditions that at least partially imitate schizophrenic behavior, one of these being manic-depression, in which the patient becomes rambling, incoherent and hallucinatory. Also Kraepelin had no biological evidence. There was nothing discernible in the blood or the saliva. He based his ideas on pure intuition, and he defended them staunchly against the outcries of nay-sayers.

One of the great distinctions Kraepelin made was that schizophrenia was a *deteriorative* illness. Other diseases might have surface similarities, but they didn't end up leaving their victims mentally impaired. Schizophrenia often does that, and with sufficient frequency that it can be called a symptom. For simplicity's sake, here is a mock "case history" that includes within its parameters many of schizophrenia's trademarks.*

We'll call our patient Bill. He is both typical and unique. He is by no means a standard by which to measure this illness, but his fictional life history does embody many of the salient features of schizophrenia.

Bill was born in 1949 to two relatively normal and well-adjusted parents. There was nothing unusual in the manner of childbirth, and his earliest years showed no abnormality. As Bill progressed through school, however, it was noted that he was unusually "sensitive." He had a hard time participating in the activities of his peers, and particularly those games that required roughness or aggressiveness. The other children considered him odd. He was not very popular with the opposite sex. His personality was shy and withdrawn, and he had a discernible tendency toward brooding and daydreaming.

Yet Bill was also bright and talented. This had been noted by many of his teachers. "If he could only adjust to the group," they would say. Bill was used to hearing that he was his own worst enemy.

The first attack came when Bill was eighteen. He was in his bedroom, lying on his bed, and he began to believe that something was wrong, that the world around him was ominously changing. The Germans have a word for this—*trema*, which is akin

---

*For the purposes of this book, I have chosen to focus on chronic schizophrenia. There are other kinds, such as acute schizophrenia, which strike without warning, then disappear.

to stagefright. It is an eerie feeling of dissociation, of being out of place with the order of the universe.

Bill's first reaction was to try to get hold of himself. He realized quite acutely that there was something wrong with him, that all of his endeavors, all of his talents, were getting him nowhere in relation to other people. "There is something wrong with me!" it dawned on him. "I am sick, or ugly, or morally inferior. Perhaps it's my nose! My fingers! My penis!" He took off his clothes and examined himself critically.

To overcome whatever was wrong with him, Bill embarked on a program of self-improvement. It was an exacting program, inhumanly compulsive, and he noted it all down in a diary like the following:

Time	Activity
7:00–8:00	cold shower, toiletries, dress
8:00–8:15	encyclopedia (memorize three facts)
8:15–8:30	handwriting
8:30–8:45	jog
8:45–9:00	cold shower
9:00–9:15	vegetarian breakfast
9:15–10:00	hearing, sight, and scent exercises

And so on.

Bill found himself getting irritable and depressed. He began examining his body more closely. Was he wrong, or was his penis shriveling? He was convinced it was—and that girls probably knew this. His thoughts became more frenetic, disjointed. His mind began to accelerate dramatically. His life became like a fast-moving dream, everything flashing with extreme rapidity.

Soon after that the voices started. At first they had a slight remnant of logic. He would see people standing a hundred yards away, and he would swear he could hear every word they were saying. They were always talking about him, of course. They seemed to be telling him what to do. Eventually, however, there were just voices—chiding, jeering, laughing, criticizing him. He became deathly afraid of the television set. He was convinced the actors could actually see *him*. When Walter Cronkite came on at seven, he was looking at Bill and broadcasting secrets about him.

Soon life itself took on arcane meanings. He would see a bus driver tip his hat. This meant that the bus driver knew about Bill's penis and was secretly communicating to women shoppers. He would pick up a pencil with a broken point. The broken point had enormous significance. It meant something terrible was about to happen, probably fatal and probably by nightfall. Traditional logic became replaced by syllogisms. "Jesus' mother was a virgin," Bill might reason. "I've heard of Jesus, and I'm a virgin, so that must mean that I am Jesus' mother."

Usually it is at this point that a psychiatrist steps in. Bill's friends and family have become increasingly alarmed. They have tried to tell themselves that it will probably pass, but with each new day Bill's condition is deteriorating. The psychiatrist is confronted with a frightening spectacle. Bill is incoherent; it is impossible to talk to him. Often he sits and stares at a wall. When he does try to talk, it comes out jibberish.

Several things might be noted at this point. In a couple of ways Bill is still "the same person." He is still a person out of step with the world, albeit now he is far more dramatically so. Also he is still a very gentle person. Indeed, his fear of violence has become pathological. Now even such things as a broken pencil point have become charged with a violence of enormous proportions.

Some years ago, back in the early seventies, Hollywood made a movie called *They Might Be Giants*. The hero of the movie was a renegade mental patient who was convinced that he was really Sherlock Holmes incarnate. Holmes, of course, could take the slightest clue and find evidence of a sinister plot afoot. The dust on a shoe or the hair on a lapel was evidence of foul play by Professor Moriarty. This is the way schizophrenics may see things. Sometimes there are overlays of paranoia, but there are usually delusions of external forces that are manipulating and controlling the victim's thought processes.

Another common symptom is what we call *blunted affect*. The patient seems to lose emotional vitality. He may talk of something that would normally be horrifying to him, yet he will sound as if he

140

were reciting from a laundry list. Conversely, at other times he may show emotion, but it won't be in reaction to anything appropriate. He may see a light bulb or a fly on the wall and break into giggles or paroxysms of laughter.

We have already talked about manic-depressives. Manic-depressives may act like schizophrenics. They may have trouble communicating, they may hear voices, their minds may be racing in illogical thought sequences. Before lithium came along, we had a hard time telling who was manic and who was schizophrenic. Lithium became a diagnostic weapon in that it usually only works on one of these illnesses.

To help psychiatrists make the proper diagnosis, the American Psychiatric Association has laid down certain criteria that a patient must meet to be labeled schizophrenic.

1. Schizophrenic-type behavioral patterns must be exhibited for at least six months prior to the date of diagnosis, with no signs of remission or relief, no return to the premorbid mental condition.

2. There must be no sign of depression or mania. All vegetative symptoms must be completely ruled out. If there is any indication that the patient is depressed, then it is probable that the patient is not schizophrenic.

In addition there are five common signs or "omens," three of which must be present for certain diagnosis. The presence of two indicates "probable schizophrenia," but the doctor would want to run further diagnostic tests.

1. *Is the patient single?* This might seem startling, but victims of this illness are almost always single. They have little if any ability to "relate," and they lack the stability to form solid relationships.

2. *Does the patient have a poor work and social history?* Schizophrenics have a history of failure. Depressives, on the other hand, are often very successful right up to the time their illness overtakes them.

3. *Does the patient seem free of alcohol or drug abuse?* There are certain drug illnesses that resemble schizophrenia. To be

absolutely certain of the diagnosis, this factor should be checked for at least one year previously.

4. *Is there a family history of schizophrenia?* As we will soon demonstrate, genetics loom large. But it may not have shown up in any visible symptoms, so it is not a surefire basis for diagnosis.

5. *Did the illness strike before the age of 40?* Schizophrenia is a young person's disease. It usually appears in teens and young adults and very rarely strikes the mature and elderly.

These are the questions a psychiatrist must ask. Three positive answers will yield a diagnosis. Even two positive answers will be a danger signal, and the doctor will watch very closely for further signs and developments. Our young man Bill would get a score of 4. He is single, and he has had a poor social history. He shows no signs of alcohol or drug abuse, and the attacks coincided with his entering adulthood.

The only factor not immediately apparent is a family history of similar behavior. But we are reasonably certain, beyond scientific doubt, that schizophrenia has a genetic factor.

Freud considered schizophrenia incurable—at least within the bounds of his theories of personality. Analysis was totally ineffective, and institutionalism was medicine's only remedy. The waters grew muddied with psychosurgery, which was not a cure but a system of management. It lowered the patient's emotional level, so that the symptoms weren't quite so troublesome or frightening.

Then came the discovery of chlorpromazine, or CPZ. Young Jacques Lh., whom we mentioned on page 29, put his footprints in medicine. Within weeks of receiving an injection of chlorpromazine, he was pronounced cured and released on his own recognizance.

But was he really cured? How could we know? *Cure* is a word my profession detests. We are willing to talk about relief or remission, but to use the word *cure* calls for a dangerous assumption. CPZ met a wall of doubt. The patients seemed tranquilized; they looked zonked and zombielike. Had we really achieved a significant breakthrough, or had we only come up with a new kind of straitjacket?

It has taken years to determine the answer to this, but now we know beyond the shadow of a doubt: CPZ is not just a sedative; it is an active agent in fighting psychosis. It does not help everyone, and it does not help permanently. Schizophrenics may have periods of relapse. Nor will CPZ restore them to absolute normalcy or make them aggressive or turn them into extroverts. The patients you see who have been released from hospitals often must live in "halfway" facilities. They may be incapable of entering the job market or contributing to society as average citizens. But they *are* improved. Even if they must live in inadequate hotels, they are light-years removed from either Bedlam or Bellevue. By normal standards their lives are constricted, but at least it's a life, and that's a major step forward for them.

Because schizophrenia is such a complicated illness, it's rather hard to discuss within the confines of this chapter, so let's just look at a few isolated facts that may give you a handle on what we're talking about.

From a statistical viewpoint schizophrenia is devastating. It strikes 500,000 people in the United States annually. If you totaled all the known cases in the world today, it would equal the entire population of New York City. In 1971 some statisticians tried to estimate the cost of schizophrenia to Americans. The figure they came up with was $14 billion annually—and that's a fraction of what it would be at present inflation rates.

Schizophrenia follows set demographics. It is far more prevalent in large urban complexes. On a per-capita basis, it is a core city ailment, showing up more frequently among lower economic groups. For a long time we wondered if the illness was environmental. Was squalor or poor nutrition the triggering mechanism? We still aren't sure, but we tend to think not—we suspect that this statistic is simply a reflection of where sick people gravitate. People with problems tend to head toward the cities. They head toward areas where there are stronger support systems. In the teeming streets they find anonymity; their eccentricities are either ignored or tolerated. We see no evidence of racial factors, nor are there any remarkable gender distinctions. Around the world and in every society, men and women seem equally afflicted by it.

While schizophrenia is always schizophrenia, it can be colored by history and environment. Today's schizophrenics talk differently from yesterday's, and midwesterners don't act the same as easterners. Most schizophrenics think they are being controlled, but the means of that control change from era to era. In the Middle Ages they thought the devil had hold of them, and there were many ecclesiastics who were willing to agree with that. In the nineteenth century the "villains" changed perceptibly. Witchcraft gave way to electricity and mesmerism. The modern schizophrenic blames TV and X-rays and is more likely to feel controlled by "outer-space radar signals."

In one of the more interesting studies of geographical influences, schizophrenics in Kentucky were matched with those in New York hospitals. The former were found to be far less communicative and far less likely to admit what was troubling them. New Yorkers, on the other hand, were much more voluble, although this did not result in their making more sense. (I suspect that there might be many in this country who would hold the same opinion of the Big Apple's nonpsychotics.) In general, as urbanization creeps in, catatonia gives way to volubility and loquaciousness. Interestingly, too, the modern schizophrenic is less likely to become violent or submit to rages.

One of the more convenient aspects of evolution is that it tends to weed out the genetically handicapped. By making the victim either deformed or asocial, there is far less chance that the strain will be propagated. Up until recently it has been that way with schizophrenics. Historically, they have almost always died childless. This, however, is being reversed, and it's one of the more troubling aspects of our success in drug therapy. By present estimates, since the

144

advent of psychopharmaceuticals, the schizophrenic birth rate has climbed precipitously. More schizophrenic patients have been able to marry, and they are propagating themselves on a par with healthy people. Since we are reasonably certain that this disease is genetic, this may not bode well for the future.

These are just a few of the many, many facets of this most stubborn and intractible of mental illnesses. It is a medical problem, a social problem, a problem that touches the lives of all of us. Yet all these negatives notwithstanding, the progress we have made is truly astonishing. I would venture to say that there is not another field of medicine in which investigators have made such remarkable headway against such an implacable adversary.

Until the development of "major tranquilizers," there was hardly a form of torture that was not tried as treatment for schizophrenia. We used electroshock, exorcism, douses in ice water. We analyzed, lobotomized, rationalized and tranquilized, and absolutely nothing had any effect. Schizophrenia was truly the equivalent of cancer. It was dark, unknowable, frightening, inexorable. But now not only do we have ways of controlling it—we are beginning to think we know some of its causes.

What Causes Schizophrenia?

Our knowledge of the causes of schizophrenia—what in medical vocabulary is called the *etiology*—owes its existence to the use of drugs, which have helped us eliminate many blind alleyways. I have already mentioned lithium, of course, but two other drugs play an important role: One is, quite naturally, CPZ; the other is the drug group we call amphetamines.

Amphetamines are commonly called uppers. They make people excited and mentally alert. They also have an unusual effect on animals, causing peculiarly patterned, or "stereotyped," behavior. When an amphetamine is given to a laboratory mouse, the mouse will run around in circles and begin sniffing and scratching. Even when it is injected with a barbiturate or a sedative, this unusual behavior pattern will not be eliminated.

Once chlorpromazine was discovered, it became a very hot research item. Like all new drugs that have a seemingly high efficacy, CPZ became a favorite substance for experimentation. Inevitably in the course of all this tinkering and testing, it was injected into a mouse that had been given amphetamines. Lo and behold, the mouse stopped running! The stereotyped behavior was completely eliminated!

This led to a number of suppositions. We knew that CPZ helped calm schizophrenics. Now we could see, in the behavior of laboratory animals, that it also seemed to counter the effects of amphetamines. Could it be that there was a link between the two phenomena? Could schizophrenia and amphetamines be mysteriously connected? If so, what was the means of that connection? What could the two possibly have in common?

By this time we were already deep into transmitter research, and we had studied the neural action of amphetamines. We were reasonably sure that they worked on three transmitter families— dopamine, serotonin and norepinephrine. But that was a pretty broad area to cover. Each of these three had its own distinct functions. How could we identify the specific transmitter that might be involved in schizophrenia?

Fortunately there was another drug in existence called *apomorphine*. Apomorphine is related to morphine. It is sometimes used on poisoning victims, its most dramatic effect being the induction of vomiting. We had a bit more knowledge about apomorphine. We knew that it only worked on dopamine neurons. This would make it a perfect foil, or control substance, since its specificity was already known to us.

In an attempt to zero in on the relevant transmitter, researchers replaced amphetamines with apomorphine. Again they got the same results. The mice developed a running and sniffing behavior, which was stopped when chlorpromazine was administered.

The pieces of the puzzle began to fit together. Amphetamines, in animals, created odd behavior. The way to eliminate that odd behavior was to block or reduce the activity of dopamine neurons.

If there was a tie between this behavior and schizophrenic psychosis, the operative factor might be the activity of dopamine. Increase dopamine and you will increase psychosis. Decrease dopamine and the condition will be alleviated.

You will recall that earlier I mentioned Parkinson's disease, a neural disorder that creates jerky body movements. I said that a side effect of CPZ was to create the same kind of movements in many psychotic patients. Parkinson's disease is a dopamine disorder. There is too little dopamine within the victim's nerve cells. This creates malfunctioning of the extrapyramidal tract, which are the nerves that control the fluidity of our muscle movement.

If parkinsonism can be treated with L-Dopa, the precursor that builds up dopamine in brain cells, then it stands to reason that in a schizophrenic L-Dopa would lead to heightened psychosis. And, in many instances, this is what researchers found. Parkinsonism and schizophrenia are both dopaminergic. While a reduction of dopamine seems to lead to parkinsonism, it also alleviates schizophrenia.

There are three brain areas concerned, according to this theory. All three are serviced by dopamine nerve cells. When I tell you what they are and describe their function, their role in schizophrenia will seem relatively apparent.

One is the *reticular activating system*. This is an area of the midbrain and brain stem whose function is to monitor incoming sensory data and to filter out that which is superfluous to the organism.

The second is the area that was discovered by Papez. We described it earlier as the *limbic system*, the brain's emotional coloring plant, the area that matches up moods to thought processes.

The third is the *hypothalamus*, which controls responses to stimuli. It works through the pituitary and endocrine system and influences the activity of the autonomic nervous system.

Now let's go back to our "case history" of Bill. We described him as experiencing a sped-up thought process. The world seemed to be coming at him fast and furious, and his consciousness was

147

reeling in sensory confusion. This could indicate a problem in the functioning of his reticular activating system. Somehow the filtering process may have collapsed. Through an overactivation of the nerves in this brain area, the most insignificant details took on added importance to him.

Second, we talked about inappropriate affect. We said that schizophrenics may laugh when nothing is funny. We said that they might talk about the most tragic experience and yet show none of the emotion we consider an appropriate reaction. This could be the result of a malfunction in the limbic system. The limbic system controls our moods and emotions. If something goes wrong in the nerve tracts in this area, it is reasonable to assume that our moods may be affected by it.

Last, we talked about a host of responses that included various abnormal body sensations. These might come from the hypothalamus, whose role is crucial in governing our hormonal responses.

Taken together, these pieces form a picture, and at the center of that picture is the chemical *dopamine*. A defect or malfunction in the creation of that chemical could lead to the illness we call schizophrenia.

Neurotransmitters are created by cells. Cells, in turn, are genetically programmed. Therefore, if schizophrenia is cellular, it would help to know if the disease is inherited.

The Genetic Factor

The suspicion that schizophrenia is an inherited disease has been around since the time of the ancient Greeks. When they weren't blaming the illness on the gods or the Furies, they were usually saying that it was a weakness in the bloodline. This suspicion endured into the twentieth century. Even Freudianism couldn't quite eradicate it. Not until the advent of drugs, however, and the resultant emphasis on biochemistry did science bring empiricism to bear on the problem.

In a remarkable study during the 1960s, Drs. Seymour Kety and David Rosenthal led a team of researchers to Copenhagen, Denmark, to search for the genetic link to schizophrenia. The researchers' reasoning went like this: Studies of twins and other unadopted children too often left open the question of environment—was schizophrenia inherited or a matter of upbringing? But what if you could find a group of adopted schizophrenics, all of whom had been raised by nonblood relatives, then go back and examine the natural parents and see if they too had the same psychosis? It was a brilliant idea—but difficult to achieve. Where would one find such convenient guinea pigs? Not in America, where such records aren't kept. You would need a modern, homogeneous, computerized welfare state.

Fortunately such a society exists in Scandinavia, where everything is socialized. All births, all illnesses, all adoptions, all hospital records have been duly recorded in computerized control centers. Denmark was picked as an ideal location. They had all the information a psychiatrist could want. If there was a genetic factor in schizophrenia, it would surely show up in the archives in Copenhagen.

Between 1963 and 1968 the researchers scrutinized the records of more than 5,000 adopted people. Of these they learned that 507 had at one time been admitted to mental institutions. They set up a "blind" panel of independent raters who examined their records for probable schizophrenia. They also set up a control group of "normal" adoptees, matched by age, sex and social status.

It was the perfect prototype of sound methodology. Nothing was left to coincidence or bias. At no time did anybody who did any of the rating know who were the controls or who the schizophrenics. All the adoptive parents were examined; then the records of the natural parents were scrutinized. Here are the results as Kety reported them in a monograph that has had far-reaching significance:

A total of 512 relatives [of both schizophrenic and control groups] were identified through the population records; of these, 119 had died and 29 had emigrated or disappeared. There was a highly significant difference in the death rates between the biological relatives of schizophrenics (35) and the biological relatives of controls (13). That difference is probably accounted for by suicide and accidental and other traumatic deaths.

149

Of the remaining 360 relatives, more than 90 percent participated in an exhaustive psychiatric interview conducted by a Danish psychiatrist who did not know the relationship of any parent to a child. Practically all of the biological relatives themselves did not know of the relationship and so did not inform the examiner. Extensive summaries of these interviews were then prepared and edited to remove any clues that would permit guessing the relationship of the parent to a child; they were then read independently by three raters, each of whom recorded his best psychiatric diagnosis for each subject from a list of possible diagnoses ranging from "no mental disorder" to "chronic schizophrenia." After that, a consensus was arrived at among the raters, the code was broken, and the subjects were allocated to their proper roles.

It was found that, with regard to mental illness other than schizophrenia, relatives of schizophrenics do not differ from the rest. But with regard to schizophrenia, they show a higher incidence of the illness. For chronic schizophrenia the prevalence in the biological relatives of schizophrenics is 2.9 percent (five of 173 relatives) compared with 0.6 percent in the other categories combined (two of 339 relatives). . . . For . . . [all categories] of schizophrenic illness, the prevalence in those genetically related to schizophrenics is 13.9 percent compared to 2.7 percent in their adoptive relatives, or 3.8 percent in all subjects not genetically related to a schizophrenic. This speaks for the operation of genetic factors in the transmission of schizophrenia.*

While the figures may seem small to the average reader, an actuary could tell you that they are statistically startling. The genetic concordance of schizophrenia is about four times greater than where there is no blood relationship.

Today we believe that it is safe to say that genetics play a role in *all* schizophrenia—that schizophrenia, as classically defined, cannot be contracted without an inheritance factor. This inheritance factor may be great or small. It seems to involve the dopamine-

*From "Recent Genetic and Biochemical Approaches to Schizophrenia" by Seymour S. Kety, *Drug Treatment of Mental Disorders* (Raven Press).

transmitter neurons. Some imbalance of these neurons or some influence on these neurons seems to predispose a person to schizophrenia.

The Megavitamin Theory

So far we have begun with a drug that "cures" schizophrenia and gone on to discover that both dopamine and genetics seem to be intimately involved in whatever it is we're curing. Along the trail there have been many blind alleys. Normally these would be forgotten and buried. But there was one long blind alley that seems worthy of mention, if for no other reason than the publicity surrounding it.

In 1952 a scientist named J. Harley-Mason put forth a hypothesis that startled our profession: He conjectured that a process called *methylation* might somehow be involved in schizophrenia. Harley-Mason was impressed by the fact that many hallucinogens were substances that had undergone a methylating process. One in particular, a hallucinogen called *mescaline,* was similar in structure to methylated dopamine.

Mescaline, of course, had been around for years. It comes from the root of a cactus called peyote. The Indians of Mexico and the American Southwest had seemed almost to worship it as though it were a deity. It entered science in 1896 when a man named Arthur Heffter first isolated it from the cactus. It was then taken up by men like Havelock Ellis, who became fascinated with its powers and its religious significance.

In 1953 Aldous Huxley joined the bandwagon. He had been reading some articles on schizophrenia. These articles postulated, à la Harley-Mason, that schizophrenia and mescaline might somehow be related to each other. The following year Huxley published a book in which he undertook to describe his experiences with mescaline. The book was called *The Doors of Perception,* and it was to become a harbinger of the Timothy Leary period.

It was not very hard back in 1953 to make romantic leaps

between genius and insanity. If there was a provable link between psychosis and chemistry, might not the use of such chemicals open new worlds of consciousness to us? Moreover, might not psychosis be a virtue? Might it not unlock the worlds of mystics and visionaries? Who was to say that the inmates in our mental hospitals might not share the truths of William Blake or St. Augustine?

Unfortunately, back then we had yet to do our homework. We had not carefully evaluated the experience of schizophrenia. It was enough to think that these people "saw the world differently"— that they were keener, more sensitive, more perceptive than their fellow humans. This lured Huxley into some far-out theorizing. He took some mescaline and went on a "head trip." He saw many strange and wonderful colors, and he experienced fascinating changes in both temporal and spatial relationships.

By now we know that in fact schizophrenics do not usually experience such wonderful visions. They do not generally see things in brighter colors, and they do not have more insight into the nature of the universe. When schizophrenics experience hallucinations, they are rarely visual and almost always auditory. They hear voices over which they have no control, and they have a tremendous sense of frustration and powerlessness. There is nothing romantic about such a state. The average schizophrenic is troubled and agitated. Most schizophrenics experience a sense of relief and a newfound tranquility after being on a drug program.

But thirty years ago we had yet to learn this. Schizophrenia was an oyster that had yet to be opened. This led to many radical hypotheses, some of which were almost dazzling in their inventiveness. It was said that schizophrenics had an unusual odor, so their sweat was examined for exotic substances. We looked at their urine, their feces, the food they ate, hoping to come up with something strange and miraculous. And we pored over drugs— LSD and mescaline, those bizarre elixirs with such mind-warping powers—hoping against hope that within some schizophrenic's body we would find a similar substance that was affecting his cognitive powers.

This search involved some very fine scientists—men like J. R. Smythies and Humphrey Osmond and Abram Hoffer. Later, tangentially, it would involve Linus Pauling, and it would give birth to a whole new offshoot of medicine. I am not ashamed to say that I, too, was involved. I also spent time in search of the "human hallucinogen." It was one of the nobler pursuits of science at that time, its only liability being the fact that it was erroneous.

Here, briefly summarized, was the trail we were barking down:

One of the many things that goes on in our bodies is a chemical process called *methylation*, in which a nonmethyl substance becomes attracted and bound to a molecule of the methyl family. As I mentioned before, it was postulated that certain neurotransmitters, if submitted to the process of methylation, would come out having a chemical structure rather suspiciously similar to the structure of mescaline.

It was also determined that there was a substance in our body— S-adenosylmethionine—that acted as a "methyl donor," contributing to the process of methylation. Aside from this, there were "methyl collectors"—substances with an inherent attraction for methyl groups. One of these was *nicotinic acid*, also known as *niacin*.

What if the cause of schizophrenia was that the methyls were being attracted to dopamine? What if they created a new kind of compound whose psychic effect was like that of mescaline? Would it not make sense to inject nicotinic acid, or a vitamin cousin in the niacin family, and have these compete with the dopamine transmitters in attracting and binding to the villainous methyl molecules? Researchers decided that this was a line of research worth pursuing. There was nothing harmful about a methylated vitamin. It would simply compete with and cheat the dopamine transmitter, and it would be excreted harmlessly through the patient's urinary system.

The first experiments with these "methyl collectors" were performed in Saskatchewan by Humphrey Osmond and Abram Hoffer, both sound scientists with impressive credentials. They administered doses of nicotinic acid to a number of patients with psychotic disorders. When they collected the results, their findings were astounding—they had "improved" 70 percent of the schizophrenics!

This set off a wave of similar experiments. New hypotheses

153

began to crop up in literature. One of these concerned a substance called *adrenochrome,* which was also considered hallucinogenic. Adrenochrome had been known for years and was often used by dentists to stop patients from hemorrhaging. But now, in the onrush of new discoveries, it was thought that it might also be found in brain tissue.

To alter the supposed effects of adrenochrome, it was proposed that vitamin C should be administered. So, along with nicotinic acid, patients were also put on a vitamin-C regimen.

And then, of course, there was LSD—lysergic acid diethylamide. This had been discovered in 1938 and was known to have powerful hallucinogenic properties. LSD is called an *indol* substance. Indol substances are chemically related to serotonin. We have internally produced indols in our bowels and in our feces, so it was not totally improbable that there might be a connection somewhere. Perhaps schizophrenics, through some quirk of nature, were absorbing indols into their brain systems. Perhaps these, in the way we supposed LSD to work, were either increasing or decreasing their neurotransmitter activity.

So there was a tremendous amount of scientific activity concerning these various substances and their relation to schizophrenia. This research would extend over the next two decades and would spawn a new school called *orthomolecular psychiatry* that would lean heavily on vitamins and dietary supplements in treatments. Even when the results were less than promising, new fuel would be added by outside sources. When Linus Pauling gave his blessings to vitamin C, the orthomolecular school gained public prominence.

But consider for a moment what concrete evidence we had to go on. There was only a presumptive connection between mescaline and dopamine. We had the unexamined notion that a hallucinogenic would create the same effect as schizophrenia. We had an unproven theory about a chemical called adrenochrome. We had even more unproven notions about LSD. And we had an unverified report from two doctors in Canada that schizophrenics had responded to vitamin therapy. What we had created for ourselves was a primrose path, and gladly, energetically, we led ourselves down it. It was so compellingly logical, so alluringly probable, that to this day there are some who have refused to abandon it.

To examine these precepts one by one: if there exists such a thing as an internally produced mescaline, it must be shown that there is something in the chemistry of schizophrenics that makes it different from other people's. Thirty years later this has yet to be proved. In fact, if anything our experiments have proved the opposite. There is not a single substance in the body of a schizophrenic that cannot also be found in many normal people.

Hallucinogens do *not* mimic schizophrenia. Schizophrenia is *not* like a mescaline or an LSD trip. In fact, the only condition that comes close to schizophrenia is the psychosis that sometimes results from amphetamines.

The adrenochrome hypothesis was a total washout. We have proved beyond a doubt that it is not in our bodies. It has yet to be found by the most sophisticated detection systems, including gas chromotography and mass spectroscopy. In fact, we have never found any internally produced hallucinogen that we could reasonably suspect produces schizophrenia. And, even if some substances might be hallucinogenic, they seem also to exist in normal people.

Finally, what about those reports from Canada? Wouldn't an improvement rate of 70 percent among schizophrenics indicate that megavitamins might indeed be worth trying?

It is important to put the answer to that in context. The human organism is extremely complicated. There are many things that might cause psychosis, including, at least remotely, dietary deficiencies. I shall not deny that some schizophrenics may have benefited from vitamin therapy. The chances that this improvement was physiologically induced are extremely slim, but even that is a possibility. Nevertheless, as a scientific therapy, the administration of vitamins is empirically invalid. You can feed all the niacin you want to mental patients, and at the end of the year, you will not have diminished your case load.

The reason the Canadian study was misleading is that it was not conducted with "double blind" safeguards. The only control was the use of placebo, but the doctors involved knew the identity of the control group. Given the general enthusiasm and optimism of that period, it is not surprising that the vitamins worked wonders. They were *supposed* to work wonders. We had high expectations for them, and those expectations were probably transmitted to the mental patients. It is now decades later, and in all these years we have yet to substantiate those original test results. We are now quite certain that they will never be substantiated because there is no medical value in vitamin therapy.

Nevertheless, because vitamins are "healthy," a small cult has sprung up of orthomolecular therapists. Its members run the gamut from accredited psychiatrists to semi-trained psychologists and blatant con artists, who remain convinced that nutrients are the key. These therapists take samples of hair. They analyze these samples and pronounce the cause of the problem to be a deficiency in zinc or some other substance. And who am I to say that they will invariably be wrong? Although their chances of helping people are virtually negligible, a suffering person will grasp at straws, particularly when the straw appears as harmless as a vitamin regimen.

In the case of Bill, if we were to give him niacin, there might be one chance in a thousand that his condition would respond to it. You would not accept such odds at Las Vegas or Hialeah, and I see no reason to accept them when being treated by psychiatrists. Perhaps the most telling proof of the failure of megavitamin therapy is that the doctors who still champion it now also prescribe tranquilizers. They combine the vitamins with antipsychotics, then point with pride to the wonderful results they achieve. If you were to go to an internist with a serious infection and he administered leeches with an antibiotic, it would be possible to claim, on the basis of your recovery, that it was the leeches, not the pills, that were responsible for the success of the therapy. And there is the infinitessimal chance that this assumption may be correct. We do not know enough about individual differences. But you would be right to denounce that internist as a quack for having the temerity to suggest such an outlandish hypothesis.

Therefore let's just stick with what we know for certain: Drugs can help many schizophrenics. In Chapter 9 we'll discuss what we know about these drugs, including some features that continue to trouble us.

9

Schizophrenia II— The Almost-Miracle Drugs

By 1952 we had discovered chlorpromazine, and by 1954 it was relatively well known, yet we persisted in following other fantasies that looked simpler, neater, faster, less complicated. There was the megavitamin theory, which I have already talked about. There was the sweat-smell theory, and the feces and food theories. Another theory I particularly remember was the dialysis theory, because I was involved in it.

As I recall, the year was about 1978. There was a kidney specialist in Florida. He had put a schizophrenic patient with kidney disease on a dialysis machine and completely recycled this patient's blood. Observing the patient's mental condition, he then made note of an unusual finding. The patient was no longer raving and hallucinatory. His schizophrenia seemed to have been eliminated!

This unusual patient, whose name has been obscured, became an anonymous celebrity in many medical circles. He seemed to be the key to an interesting hypothesis—that there was some sort of link between psychosis and kidney function. What happened next was even more startling. This patient underwent a kidney transplant—and within a very short time after the operation, he relapsed back into schizophrenia!

Now here was the promise of a remarkable new breakthrough. Through the miracle of dialysis we had cured schizophrenia. Not only that but we had established a connection between the human kidney and a severe psychological disorder. Think of the wonderful possibilities. We could put all our mental patients on dialysis machines, flush their bodies at periodic intervals, and thereby end these horrible behavior problems.

Soon after word about dialysis got around, a rumor began circulating from another quarter. Another doctor, who I think should remain anonymous, announced that he had replicated the kidney specialist's discovery. He went further than that, saying that, with the help of a biochemist, he had also isolated a suspicious substance. They had analyzed the blood and found an abnormal endorphin that was undoubtedly the cause of this devastating psychosis!

I cannot tell you the excitement this created. At last we had our elusive "toxin"! The villain was no longer methylated dopamine, it was an endogenous, but structurally abnormal, painkiller!

I called this doctor, who was at one of the larger state-run medical schools. "Is it true?" I asked.

"Yes, it is," he said.

"Stay right where you are. I'm taking the next plane out," I said.

When I got there, I was greeted by an enthusiastic doctor talking glowingly about his miraculous discovery. It was going to revolutionize all of psychiatry. It was going to be bigger than the discovery of Thorazine.

"When are you going to publish?" I asked him.

"Publish? Well, yes . . . I'm planning to do that. But first I want to get some more data . . . some corroborating evidence that will make it all airtight . . ."

I decided to give him the benefit of the doubt. I knew that unpublished findings are just so much hearsay, but if he insisted on being so secretive about his findings, that was his affair, and I would just have to be patient.

In the meantime I had gathered enough scattered evidence to make his hypothesis seem worth pursuing. I requested a grant from the National Institute of Health to conduct my own experiments to try to substantiate his discovery.

The end of this story is predictable, I suppose. There was no endorphin that created psychosis. The doctor, although he may have been sincere, had gotten carried away on the wings of some fantasy. As for the kidney specialist, he was certainly genuine, but his dialysis findings have never been duplicated. They have never withstood a "double blind" test using "sham" dialysis to rule out placebo factors.

As for me? I survived. My grant was turned down—the NIH said it was all a bunch of foolishness—but, outside of having some egg on my face, I don't consider it among life's greater tragedies. If you're a scientist, you're going to be wrong sometimes. You're going to be misled. You're going to look foolish. But if you aren't willing to take that risk, you're not very likely to contribute anything. I think of Nate Kline, the man with reserpine. He has been wrong, and he has also been criticized for it. Some are envious of the fame he has accrued, and they have accused him of using too much showmanship. But Nathan Kline has been a genuine contributor. He introduced reserpine and MAO inhibitors. Compared with these, his failures seem pale. Who cares if Columbus thought America was India?

Perhaps the most remarkable thing about all these decades of theorizing is that the original discovery never lost its significance. CPZ steadily gained acceptance, and it spawned other drugs that proved somewhat superior to it.

CPZ is of a chemical family that goes under the name of *phenothiazine*. There are a number of phenothiazines around, and they have proved quite useful in this nation's therapy programs. But there are also other kinds of antipsychotics. You will find a list of them on page 161. The use of these drugs—and also their *ill* effects—has become the most dominant trademark of modern psychiatry.

Today's Antipsychotics

Looking back, most psychiatrists nowadays are sorry that we ever invented the term *major tranquilizers*. *Tranquilizers* suggest that the patient is sedated, and we now know that is not how these drugs really help people. In the early days, when Thorazine became popular, there were, unfortunately, sedative side effects. Patients would wander, dazed and inchoate, their slippered feet moving in an odd kind of shuffling manner. We also confronted other problems. One was hypotension, or low blood pressure. Another was a disturbing muscle illness called *tardive dyskenesia*, which will be discussed later.

Some of these problems were matters of procedure. We really didn't know how to use these drugs properly. We were using them as a preventative, as we now use lithium, and were administering them to patients as a daily regimen. But defects were also inherent in the medicine. Hypotension is dangerous for elderly people. And tardive dyskenesia, while it's rarely fatal, was irreversible in about half of all drug patients.

Solving these problems has been an ongoing process. I am sorry to say that some are still with us. But the progress we have made has been very encouraging, and today's schizophrenics have a lot more going for them.

In the late 1950s, a young Belgian chemist, Paul A. J. Janssen, stumbled across a substance that would have the ultimate effect of making CPZ seem old-fashioned and obsolescent. Janssen had been serving in the Belgian military, and when his tour was up he looked around for a job. His family owned a very modest chemical plant in the town of Beerse, not far from Brussels. The plant was impoverished, it owned no patents, it hardly had the means of providing an income. Nevertheless, Janssen cast his lot with it, and he gathered around him a group of young researchers.

They set to work in 1953 looking for derivatives of available chemicals. For budgetary reasons they used inexpensive chemicals, but they approached the task with naive enthusiasm. One of the first things they discovered was *diphenoxylate*. You may know it better by its trade name, Lomotil. Today it is the most famous of all anti-diarrhetics, and few visitors to Mexico have not had to resort to it.

Table 1
The Antipsychotics

Generic Name	Brand Name	Company
Phenothiazines		
Chlorpromazine	Thorazine	Smith Kline & French
Fluphenazine	Prolixin	Squibb
	Permitil	White
Mesoridazine	Serentil	Boehringer Ingelheim
Perphenazine	Trilafon	Schering
Prochlorperazine	Compazine	Smith, Kline & French
Thioridazine	Mellaril	Sandoz
Trifluoperazine	Stelazine	Smith, Kline & French
Triflupromazine	Vesprin	Squibb
Butyrophenones		
Haloperidol	Haldol	McNeil
Thioxanthenes		
Chlorprothixene	Taractan	Roche
Thiothixene	Navane	Pfizer Roerig
Indolones		
Molindone	Moban	Endo
Dibenzoxazepines		
Loxapine	Loxitane	Lederle

The second thing they came up with was *butyrophenone*. When they injected it into mice, they got an unusual reaction. They discovered that it acted somewhat like morphine, but it also had certain CPZ or tranquilizing properties. Since they did not want a tranquilizer that acted like opium, they modified it again, deemphasizing the opiate. The result was an agent called *haloperidol,* more potent than chlorpromazine, but with fewer side effects.

Today haloperidol (trade name, Haldol) is one of the leading drugs in the treatment of psychosis. It shares this distinction with Prolixin and Navane, all three of which are more popular than Thorazine. It takes 2 doses of Prolixin or Haldol to equal 100 doses of a drug like Thorazine. This means that you can have all the benefits of Thorazine without flooding the patient's system with chemicals.

More important, these newer drugs have fewer effects on the various organs. They are less sedating, they produce more alertness and they do not precipitate a decrease in blood pressure. We might call these the second-generation drugs. They are what you will usually find being used in hospitals. Stelazine is another very effective drug, but it is an older drug, and therefore less fashionable.

Besides these salutory advances in chemistry, we have also learned more about drug administration. We now know that keeping a patient sedated is not only dangerous, it is also unnecessary. In the old days, when CPZ was first used, we kept schizophrenics on unrelieved therapy. We thought that it was worth putting up with sedation to prevent the threat of a psychotic relapse. Today we employ what are called drug holidays, which relieve the patients from antipsychotics. We watch them carefully to determine their condition, and only as they worsen do we put them on drugs again.

Nevertheless, despite these improvements, there are still some aspects that are unappealing. One of these is the extrapyramidal syndrome, which, although it is not serious, is still a drawback.

Extrapyramidal Effects

Earlier in this book we described the extrapyramidal tracts, which help control fluidity of movement. These are nerve tracts which originate below the cortex, and are under the control of dopamine neurons. When you deplete the dopamine, the tracts malfunction. This creates a jerky body movement of the sort one sees in victims of parkinsonism.

Antipsychotics are dopamine blockers. They block the dopamine at the postsynaptic-receptor site. This sometimes leads to a kind of pseudoparkinsonism, a jerky movement that can be alarming to patients' relatives.

I want to stress that these cases are infrequent. Most of our patients suffer no such side effects. But they do show up on a regular-enough basis that they are considered common within the context of drug therapy. The important thing to remember is that these extrapyramidal effects are usually temporary and will disappear. In fact, our preference is to do nothing about them—let the body adapt and let nature do its healing work.

In case the symptoms grow too severe, or in the event that they continue beyond a reasonable period, we do have drugs that are very effective in controlling extrapyramidal effects. One of these is Artane, and two other drugs often used are Cogentin and Kemadrin. We have even obtained satisfactory results with antihistamines, like the popular Benadryl. These drugs do not work on the dopamine neurons. Remember: Elevated dopamine increases psychosis. What these drugs do is work indirectly—they decrease the activity of an *opposing* neuronal system.

You will recall that our nerves are like a system of government—everything works by checks and balances. When you decrease one network another accelerates. It is the lack of equilibrium that results in side effects.

The neurons opposing dopamine neurons are a family of nerve cells containing acetylcholine. When dopamine goes down, acetylcholine goes up. When you decrease acetylcholine activity, you help control parkinsonism.

Think of it like this:

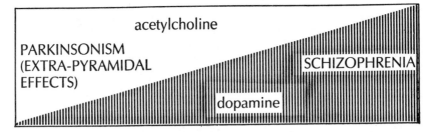

The trouble is that when you decrease acetylcholine and allow the dopamine to reassert itself, you are also taking a calculated risk that you might bring back the symptoms of schizophrenia. This is why, except in dire cases, we would prefer not to use an anticholinergic drug and continue use of the antipsychotic in the hopes that parkinsonism will remit spontaneously.

The extrapyramidal effects of these drugs, while briefly alarming if you are visiting a loved one, are not really very serious and certainly no reason to grow concerned or fearful. Far more disturbing is tardive dyskenesia. This is a number-one medical priority. Fortunately it too has become more manageable, but it is still awaiting a major breakthrough.

Tardive Dyskenesia

In the early days of drug therapy, we administered massive doses of Thorazine. In the schizophrenic wards of our large state hospitals, patients wandered about in a tranquilized daydream. Then one day we noticed something peculiar. Some patients developed a strange, wormlike tongue movement. It was hardly noticeable—a twitch of the tongue tip—but you could see it when they held their mouths open. As the days passed by, the symptoms grew worse. Their lips began rotating in a chewing movement. Soon the whole mouth was thrusting and rolling, the tongue flicking out like the tongue of an anteater.

What kind of strange behavior was this? It grew worse. It afflicted their arms and legs. They began to writhe slowly, purposelessly, a few of them developing a to-and-fro rocking motion.

Little did we know it, but we were in the process of observing the first serious drawback of antipsychotics. It came to be known as delayed abnormal muscle reaction—or, in medical terms, *tardive dyskenesia*. It swept through the hospitals like an epidemic. One after another the patients were stricken. Soon we had almost 50 percent of our mental patients chewing and grimacing in a horrible grotesquerie.

What was the cause? We didn't know. Families of the afflicted patients went running to the doctors. "What have you done to poor Joe?" they demanded. "He's writhing so badly, we can't stand the sight of him!"

Well, what we had done was try to fool nature—and nature, as usual, was not cooperating. It had grown used to those higher dopamine levels, and it was finding new ways to get around Thorazine. The Thorazine, you see, was blocking the receptors. The receptors were not getting their usual transmitter messages. They were being required to fire less often, and it was a state of lethargy they were not accustomed to.

Nature does not adapt well to change. It finds new ways of behaving as it always did. So when the patient's body found that dopamine was being short-circuited, it simply instructed the receptors to become more sensitive. They began to fire on fewer transmitters, sending out ill-conceived impulses to various body parts. Worse than that, new receptors appeared. The postsynaptic neurons grew abnormally sensitive.

Thus antipsychotics can be sorcerers' apprentices. The harder they work, the more their work is cut out for them. Soon they are faced with multiple dopamine receptors, each determined to keep up the firing activity.

The tragedy in this is that the damage is often permanent. The new receptors cannot be easily demolished. This, of course, leads to irreversible symptoms—a muscular condition that is unacceptable.

So far we have yet to solve this conundrum, which has become the most nagging problem in psychopharmacology. We are still struggling with certain "halfway" procedures—procedures that help but are by no means adequate.

One positive factor is that since we know what to look for, and since we are acutely aware of the implications, hospital staffs and even nonmedical health workers are much more alert to the earliest signs of tardive dyskenesia. As soon as they see those telltale tongue movements, they alert the psychiatrist or physician in charge. Medication is immediately stopped, and the illness is checked or brought into remission. The doctor then faces a critical choice: Which is worse, the psychosis or the muscle movements? Should he go back to the drug, risking dyskenesia, or should he allow the return of the previous mental condition?

Quite frankly, this is a hell of a choice. The patient is likely to be happier on the drug, but the tics and writhings may be so unsightly that even her fellow patients can't stand to look at her. Ironically, there is a way to stop this—increase the dosage of the drug that caused it. Unfortunately this is only a delaying tactic, and a potentially dangerous one. Since the condition is caused by sensitized dopamine receptors plus the stimulated growth of additional receptors, it stands to reason that if you step up the drug you can temporarily inhibit this increased sensitivity. It also stands to reason that it may not stay inhibited. Nature again may frustrate your purposes. To make matters worse, you might create still more receptors, and so on, until you have created a debacle.

Ultimately we must find a true antidote, some drug that will stop or prevent dyskenesia. There are three possibilities that come to mind, and we are hoping that one of them is the answer we're looking for.

1. *Go back to using reserpine.* This would be an unusual twist. Reserpine, you'll recall, created depression and was a negative impetus in the development of drug therapy. But since reserpine decreases storage of dopamine transmitters, it may be helpful in preventing dyskenesia.

2. *Use lithium to help block excess receptor formation.* This, too, is a promising line of research. So far it seems to work well in animals, but its use in humans remains theoretical.

3. *Introduce an agent that increases acetylcholine.* One such agent is *lecithin,* which is produced within the body and can also be found in a variety of foodstuffs. Lecithin is a very interesting chemical, and we'll be talking about it again in our chapter on diet. It is a *lipotropic*—that is, it metabolizes fats—and it may play a role in our higher brain functions.

Lecithin contains a substance called *choline*. Choline is a "precursor" of acetylcholine. If you can get large amounts of the stuff into mental patients, this might help offset the effects of the dopamine.

These are the three key areas of research, and we are hoping that one will lead to a breakthrough. In the meantime we are operating on improved drug management, which is at least holding the line against this troublesome side effect.

One possible consolation is that only a minority of patients get tardive dyskenesia. I would estimate that the percentage affected is significantly below what it was twenty years ago. We have reason to believe that the patients who do get it usually fall into one of four categories.

1. patients who have been on antipsychotics for years
2. patients who have had a history of alcohol abuse
3. patients who have had an abnormally high number of shock treatments
4. elderly patients with other kinds of brain damage

All four are related to some form of brain damage, and realizing this has been a major help to us.

Although tardive dyskenesia is an unpleasant problem, it should not be allowed to alarm the patient. For friends and relatives the primary concern should be that their loved one is being treated adequately for his psychosis.

Odds and Ends

This completes our section on the treatment of various illnesses. I have tried to make it as complete as the limits of space allow. Needless to say, it is not comprehensive, there being so many types and subtypes of illnesses. There are, for example, two serious ailments which are very rare, but may be of interest.

GILLES DE LA TOURETTE'S DISEASE

In 1885 Gilles de la Tourette published a description of a most unusual psychopathology: he had a patient who barked, had a number of body tics and was given to outbursts of the most astonishing invective! We named this condition after the man who described it. I am happy to say that it is very, very rare, and when it does show up, we have a drug that manages it.

The classic definition of Gilles de la Tourette's disease is that it usually first appears among very young children. It generally shows up before the age of twelve, manifesting itself in the most hideous body tics. The patient begins with spasmodic grimacing. Soon the entire upper body is involved. Eventually he may begin hopping and skipping, expressing himself through various odd motor movements.

But the symptom that draws the most attention is the incessant string of four-letter words. The victim will spit, cough, bark like a dog, then let you have it with an outburst of gutter talk!

We really aren't sure what causes this. We believe it's related to dopamine-transmitter neurons. We also know that the children who have it are usually male and may have parents with paranoid symptoms.

For years we were stumped as to what treatment to use. Nothing seemed to have any effect. We tried insulin, hypnosis, electroshock, reconditioning therapy—nothing seemed to be very effective against it.

Then, by happy coincidence, along came *haloperidol,* which, you'll recall, is an antipsychotic discovered by Janssen and his co-workers and now used frequently in place of Thorazine. Dr. Arthur K. Shapiro of Mt. Sinai Hospital found that if you put a patient on haloperidol, he will begin to calm down and act more normally. After a year or so of heavy treatment, there will be a 90-percent reduction in symptoms. This is another problem for which we have found a treatment but have yet to determine what it is we're treating. Hopefully, in the years ahead the drug may lead us to the disease's origins.

PARANOIA

I suppose you may think it's a bit ironic, living as we do in the 1980s, that I would take an ailment like paranoia and dismiss it in a couple of paragraphs. Because assuredly, if there is any trademark of our times, it is the feeling that there is "someone out to get us"—the FBI, the Mafia, the Communists, even, heaven forbid, psychiatrists or drug companies! But pure paranoia is a very rare illness. More frequently it is attached to schizophrenia. We have already seen how our young friend Bill hallucinated that people on the street were saying bad things about him.

True paranoia, without schizophrenia, is what we might find embodied in people like Hitler or Stalin. It is very organized and has certain bits of logic to it, and the person who possesses it may be verbal and persuasive about it. Because the victims are more coherent and because they tend to be older, they are among the hardest patients to treat—if, indeed, you can get them to a psychiatrist's office. Paranoia takes many forms. It may be a husband who is insanely jealous. It may be a young woman, lonely and unattractive, who is convinced that one of the Beatles is secretly in love with her. Lon Chaney's *Wolfman* was a rare kind of paranoid—*lycanthropy* (the belief that one is a wolf) was recorded in the Middle Ages. There is another paranoid state that is associated with voodoo, in which a victim can actually die because of being terrorized by a witch doctor.

We try to get paranoid patients to place some modicum of trust in us. We try to use ourselves as psychic bridges, leading them back into the world of reality. Along with that we may use drug therapy, but antipsychotics are rarely effective. The road to recovery is slow and difficult, and for that reason it is fortunate that the disease is not very prevalent.

10

Your Diet and Your Brain— Some Facts, Some Fantasies

Frankly, when I was asked to compile a chapter on the contributions of diet to mood changes, I was somewhat hesitant, as most doctors would be, fearing the effects that my words might have. America has become the land of faddism. There is a percentage of the populace that acts like lemmings. As soon as they hear that something is good for you, they will run off and buy it, regardless of consequences. This has become complicated by our notions of "natural." If vitamins are "natural," then drugs must be "unnatural"—the conclusion of which is that if we load up on vitamins we will obviate the need for pharmaceuticals.

In addition, we are selectively paranoid. We believe some sources but are skeptical of others. Whom and what we choose to believe depends more on our prejudices than on logic or intellect. I am reminded of a quote that appeared recently in a newspaper concerning the attitudes and biases of American young people: "If you want to sell vitamins to this group," said a Madison Avenue executive, "use a star athlete, but not a doctor."

Well, I'm not in the business of selling vitamins, but I cling to the notion that I may have learned some things that even Bruce Jenner hasn't. I have learned, for example, that some people are afraid. Even when they are ill, they will try to avoid drugs and instead will take all kinds of worthless concoctions that are sold under the aegis of being "nature's own remedy." They have accepted the notion that the body is perfect, and if we feed it properly it will somehow correct itself. They ignore genetics. They ignore evolution. They ignore the possibility that nature has flaws.

This chapter is not addressed to these people. I doubt if they are the types who would read it anyway. They will continue to spend small fortunes on health-food products, accepting the advice of a cab driver over that of a medical doctor. Indeed, such prejudices can even be found among professionals. There have been a number of food studies that purport to be objective, blaming poor health on everything from eggs to sugar to wheat, but few, if any, stand up to scrutiny. It is not quite correct that "we are what we eat." *We are by and large what we were genetically programmed to be*. But since a small percentage is at least in our control, let's take a look at the few things we know about it.

Vitamins

Dr. Paul Greengard, a pharmacologist at Yale, has this to say about Americans' use of vitamins:

> Probably no single class of drugs has been the target of as much quackery, misunderstanding, misrepresentation, and misuse as the vitamins, despite the fact that far more is known about these compounds, including their mechanism of action, than about any other group of substances. . . . Many millions of individuals living in the United States regularly ingest quantities of vitamins vastly in excess of the Recommended Daily Dietary Allowances. In the case of the water-soluble vitamins (the vitamin B complex and vitamin C), this would seem to do little harm to the body because of the low toxicity of this class of compounds. However, such practice is

171

economically wasteful and, in some instances, causes financial hardship. . . . In the case of the lipid-soluble vitamins (vitamins A, D, E and K), the compounds accumulate in the body fat and can be toxic. The conscientious physician should assure himself that his patients are not victims of the excessive use of vitamins.

What is a vitamin? Broadly speaking, it is a substance necessary for the maintenance of life, but one not synthesized within the body, so therefore incumbent upon our dietary regimen. Most vital substances are made by our body. We make everything from glucose to cholines to cholesterol. But there are a few things that are not provided, and that means that we have to go out and forage for them. We didn't understand too much about vitamins until we realized that there were diseases that could be cured by foodstuffs. Scurvy, for example, could be cured by fruits, pellagra or beriberi by castaway rice polishings. In the late nineteenth century and into the twentieth century, the vitamins in these foodstuffs were isolated and synthesized. Since they were in our diet and were deemed to be harmless, they have escaped the control of any regulatory agency.

But the truth is, in America today, there are many people who are "vitamin abusers." They are willing to go out and spend their hard-earned money on capsules and tablets that have nothing but placebo value. This is not to say there is not a role for vitamins— they are perfectly good when taken as a "supplement." But if you think they provide "medicinal therapy," in the majority of cases that is probably imaginary.

Of course there are always exceptions to this. There are rare individuals with vitamin deficiencies. Relatively few turn up in this country, but when they do, we can usually classify them. Elderly people. They often don't eat right. They are too poor or infirm to prepare what's good for them. We have already seen how certain deficiencies can mimic the symptoms of depression in old people. Food faddists and vegetarians are another group who will sometimes abuse themselves. Remember the "macrobiotic" craze, in which some young people starved from eating nothing but brown rice and beans? And alcoholics, and people with mental

172

problems, and the occasional drug addict who's been living in the slums somewhere—but generally speaking, in the industrialized West, we find very few people who need vitamin therapy.

There is little or no evidence that any vitamin actually works wonders. One that has been purported to do so is vitamin E, which is a major item on many health counters. Vitamin E has been called the sex vitamin. It's supposed to help everything from infertility to impotence. In reality, it doesn't do any of those things, but that won't prevent some hopefuls from buying it. The reason for its reputation is that its history is connected with pregnancy in rats. It was found that rodents lacking vitamin E had a very hard time giving birth. What this has to do with sex in humans is anybody's guess—it is totally irrelevant. And since E is one of the fat-soluble vitamins, it is wise not to take more than the recommended allowances of it.

Or B_{15}. Ever heard of that one? It goes by the pseudonym *pangamic acid*. It is being touted as a miracle vitamin, good for curing everything from asthma to drug addiction. B_{15} is actually a trade name invented by the same man who gave us laetrile. He is a twice-convicted criminal named Andrew McNaughton, and he is one of the most notorious charlatans in the pseudo-nutrition field.* According to Dr. Victor Herbert, a leading hematologist and nutritionist with the Bronx VA Medical Center, B_{15} is not only worthless, it has several ingredients that can actually be harmful. One is dichloroacetate. This is a gonad poison in rats. Another is dimethylglycine, which has been shown to destroy kidneys in various animal tests.

And then, of course, there is vitamin C. Vitamin C is an essential vitamin, needed in the formation of certain substances that act as the "cement" to hold our cells together. In combination with folic acid, it also plays a role in the formation of dopamine. This means that it's part of the chemical chain that leads to the creation of an important transmitter family. It is therapeutic in

*For a fuller account of McNaughton and his run-ins with the law, see *Nutrition Cultism: Facts and Fictions* by Victor Herbert, M. D., J. D. Philadelphia: Stickley, 1980. McNaughton's convictions are for stock fraud and for conspiracy to facilitate transportation of smuggled merchandise.

treating scurvy; nevertheless, in clinical trials, we have yet to establish any psychiatric value in administering vitamin C.

When I was talking about depression in the elderly, I mentioned that there are two deficiencies that can lead to mood changes: deficiency of vitamin B_{12}, and deficiency of folic acid. Vitamin B_{12} is an interesting vitamin. It is not to be found in any plant life. Rather, it is synthesized by microorganisms that are often found in animals' intestinal tracts. Beef, for example, has vitamin B_{12}, but it is manufactured inside the cow. The bacteria in the juices of the cattle's saliva mix with the grasses it eats and synthesize the vitamin.

Strict vegetarians may have B_{12} deficiencies, since these people aren't getting the substances that have B_{12}. About the only exception are certain pod-type vegetables that carry the organisms that make this vitamin.

B_{12} deficiency can be very serious. It is the leading cause of pernicious anemia and can also create various mood disorders—confusion, poor memory, depression, ataxia. B_{12} is needed for the production of myelin, the stuff in which our neurons are sheathed. What is sometimes mistaken for senility in the aged can actually arise from destruction in the individual's nervous system, caused by a lack of this important vitamin.

Folic acid is similar to B_{12}. In fact, their histories are closely related. It took many years and many experiments to distinguish the roles each plays in anemia. Similarly, there is a close relationship between folic acid and vitamin C. Vitamin C "protects" folic acid—it guards it from destruction by oxidation. When you suffer a deficiency of folic acid, you may develop symptoms of depression and confusion. To guard against this you need yeast, liver and many of the vegetables that have high vitamin C content.

Having stressed that most "vitamin therapies" are wasteful at best and in some cases harmful, I want to talk briefly about another "vitamin" whose role in psychiatry is still very speculative. I am talking about an agent called *choline*, which is found primarily in *lecithin*. (We mentioned these in Chapter 9.) Since both of these names have been in the news of late, let's try to clarify what we really know about them.

174

Choline and the Lecithin Theory

Some time ago, in its science section the *New York Times* ran an article on "brain foods." Prominently mentioned was a nutrient called lecithin, which is concentrated in egg yolk, liver and other substances. Since then there has been an increasing demand for this magical protein. I'm not sure why people are buying it, but I can at least explain why psychiatry has become interested in it.

Lecithin is of a family called *phospholipids.* It is found in a number of animal tissues. It is also highly concentrated in egg yolk, although its purest source is probably the soybean. Lecithin is a fat. It contains stearic acid, glycerol and choline. It is this latter that has drawn the attention of researchers, particularly centered on the role it may play in memory retention.

You will recall that one of the major transmitter families is *acetylcholine,* which performs many brain functions. It is acetylcholine that opposes dopamine and therefore may figure in schizophrenia. Acetylcholine, as the name implies, is made up of choline and acetic acid. Acetic acid is an aqueous solution that is a main ingredient of household vinegar.

The importance of choline first became apparent not in the brain, but in the liver of animals. It was found that when you removed the pancreas from a dog, his liver developed signs of cirrhosis. This was correctable by a diet including lecithin. The agent responsible was found to be choline. Choline, it turned out, was very important in the breakdown of fats and carbohydrates.

Choline, strictly speaking, is not a vitamin. Vitamins are agents found only outside our bodies. Choline is also produced internally, so you can only run short of it if you lack certain other substances. This has become a big question for researchers. Can a choline-free diet create a deficiency, or does the body, which also creates its own choline, merely manufacture more to make up for the deficit?

You may observe a similarity here to the theorizing about another fatty substance, *cholesterol.* We take in cholesterol with our diet, but it is also manufactured by the body internally. That this analogy exists may be somewhat ironic, because cholesterol is also contained in egg yolk. And in recent years it has been found that cholesterol will not collect in our arteries if it is taken with lecithin.

The role of choline in psychiatry is tentative. Since we know that it is a precursor of acetylcholine, we have naturally wondered whether choline (or lecithin) might alleviate psychosis or improve people's cognitive functions. We suspect, for example, that the loss of memory—particularly as one sees it in the aged or infirm— might be attributable to the destruction of neurons containing the transmitter acetylcholine. Short-term studies seem to bolster this hypothesis. We have seen memory improvement after the ingestion of choline. We have also seen improvement of certain symptoms of mania and tardive dyskenesia.

One study, however, provides indirect evidence that choline might aid even normal people's memories. It did not involve choline itself, but an associated substance called *physostigmine*.

Physostigmine comes from the seed of a bean plant that grows beside rivers in tropical West Africa. It was originally used as a deadly poison by local tribes during trials for witchcraft. Today it is often used in insecticides, and the military has studied it for chemical warfare. But like so many poisons, it is also a medicine— it depends on the dosage and the way it is administered.

Physostigmine is an *anticholinesterase*—that is, it opposes the enzyme that breaks down acetylcholine. As such, it is analagous to an MAO inhibitor, which inhibits the enzyme that destroys certain other transmitters. By inhibiting the destroyers, you increase the transmitters. Thus the effect of physostigmine is like that of choline. Both increase transmitter activity, although they do so through very dissimilar mechanisms.

In a recent study of young adults, it was found that administering physostigmine could measurably raise the memory level of a few of these subjects for a very short time. What this means we are not really certain. A study like this is extremely "iffy." But it does seem to indicate that we have found a door that will lead to a better understanding of memory.

So where does this leave us? We have an agent called choline, which seems to help certain sick people think better. We have a "poison" from West Africa called physostigmine, which may help

176

some people remember better. Last but not least, we have a substance called lecithin, which seems to contribute to the very same process. And we find, ironically, that it is contained in egg yolk and that it may help prevent the buildup of cholesterol in our arteries.

In light of these discoveries (but also in view of what we do *not* know), I think the wisest response is to proceed with prudence. Our brain cells, after all, are not our only concern. It would be unwise to pursue improvement at the risk of abusing other organs. Perhaps it would be best to remember that the human diet is the result of centuries of evolution. We should not presume that our ancestors were fools or that they passed down customs of eating substances that are inherently harmful to us. Most of the items we eat have value. We should neither abandon them nor overindulge in them. Certainly this is true of the lipid substances, which may contain both the seeds of our health and our destruction.

Hypoglycemia, or Low Blood Sugar

Illnesses come and go, like fashions. A popular one nowadays is *hypoglycemia*. In everyday English this means "low blood sugar," and it is amazing the number of people who believe they are afflicted by it.

True hypoglycemia is a serious disorder. It usually shows up in two kinds of patients: diabetics who have overdosed on insulin, and people with insulin-secreting tumors of the pancreas. Yet I doubt if there is a psychiatrist nowadays who has not had patients come into her office—usually well educated and usually female—swearing that they have been diagnosed as hypoglycemic. They are not saying that they are diabetic, and they would be truly horrified if a tumor were mentioned. Rather, what they are saying is that they feel depressed and irritable, and they have been told that low blood sugar could be the cause of this.

True hypoglycemia, as I say, is very serious, but there is another condition, *functional hypoglycemia,* an extremely rare disorder in which low blood sugar occurs without diabetes or

177

tumor of the pancreas. The reason we have so many "hypo-glycemics" is that (1) it is easily misdiagnosed, and (2) it sounds more exotic than depression—it's comforting to know there is something physically wrong with you! But, as I mentioned in earlier chapters, depression itself can have physical origins. If you are feeling moody, it is more likely to be caused by depression than anything as rare as hypoglycemia.

Nevertheless, are there hypoglycemics? A few. And they do manifest unusual mood symptoms. Here, in very ordinary language, is a thumbnail sketch of functional hypoglycemia:

When a person eats sugar—say a sweetmeat or candy bar—he is really eating *glucose*. Glucose is simply crystallized sugar, the same stuff you get in honey or fruit juice. When glucose is ingested, it must be metabolized. This is done by insulin. Insulin, as you know, is secreted by the pancreas, and in particular a section called the islets of Langerhans. In diabetics there is a bodily malfunction, and the insulin is not secreted on cue. This means that the glucose is not metabolized but passes out of the body leaving the victim in a state of "starvation."

The pancreas is part of the endocrine system. There are hormones that control the release of insulin. These hormones, in turn, are controlled by the brain, and specifically certain areas that are close to the limbic system.

When you take in glucose, two things happen—your sugar level goes up, and you start secreting insulin. The insulin quickly increases the body's utilization of glucose, and your blood-sugar level drops back to the normal range. But in a hypoglycemic something goes wrong. The insulin starts flowing, but it doesn't shut off again. It keeps metabolizing glucose without shutting off, plummeting the sugar level to the dangerously subnormal range.

When this starts to happen, the body sounds an alarm. A message is flashed to the adrenal medulla. The adrenal medulla controls the release of adrenaline, a powerful mood changer with many emergency functions. The brain has been warned that there is a falloff in blood sugar. It sends out adrenaline, which activates the liver. The liver is where starch is stored. The liver "chops off" the starch into little links of glucose.

The result is a runaway chemical action. The liver is producing glucose to elevate the sugar, but the pancreas is continuing to pour out insulin, and the adrenal medulla is still secreting adrenaline. In terms of mood, here's what this means: The variances in blood sugar may make you depressed. This feeling initially is usually mild and will not create profound or startling behavioral changes. But when the blood sugar continues to drop, sending an alarm to your adrenal medulla, the adrenaline that this gland pumps through your system can have very profound and startling effects. Adrenaline is similar to norepinephrine. It can create more powerful mood changes than a drop-off of blood sugar. You can become depressed, anxious, irritable, nervous. This may compel you to see a psychiatrist.

A good psychiatrist, who is alert to this problem, will ask you questions such as the ones that appear on page 86. He will be looking closely for "vegetative symptoms," and he will be particularly interested in the pleasures you are experiencing. You see, hypoglycemics are not really depressives. The true depressive does not know pleasure. The hypoglycemic *does* find pleasure, but it may be obscured or obstructed by feelings of misery.

Why is this illness so popular right now? For one thing, it is often misdiagnosed. Many MDs mistakenly believe low blood-sugar levels to be an adequate reason for diagnosis. Low blood sugar is only one of the symptoms, and it must be extraordinarily low for hypoglycemia to be present. Relatively low levels will not alarm your body and send adrenaline racing throughout the bloodstream.

Nevertheless, once in a great while we will find a patient with hypoglycemia, and this is raising some interesting questions about the origins and pathways of this peculiar condition. It is commonly supposed that the cause must be physical: There may be something organically wrong with the pancreas, or there may be something wrong with the nerves and regulators whose job it is to turn off the production of insulin. But what if we turned the question around? What if we applied the James-Lange hypothesis (see p. 59)? Is it not possible that low blood sugar might actually be created by *psychic* disturbances?

179

If you look at the mechanism, the potential is there. Insulin is regulated by a confluence of other hormones. One of these is called growth hormone (GH), and the other is called somatostatin. These are produced by the pituitary gland and an adjoining structure, the hypothalamus. These are related to the limbic system, which is the "coloring plant" for much of our emotional life.

This has led scientists to the speculation—and I stress that it is *only* a speculation—that the insulin malfunction in hypoglycemia may in fact be *caused* by one's moods or emotionalism. This would be an interesting phenomenon. It would mean that a physical malfunction that affects one's psyche could be caused by the very same psyche, creating a cyclical condition that is self-exacerbating. As a relay station between our body and our thoughts, the limbic system can turn abstractions into chemistry. Are our hormones making us moody, or is it our moods that are affecting our hormones? No one knows—but it's an interesting problem.

At present the usual remedy for hypoglycemia is physical. We try to moderate glucose intake so as not to set off a wild rush of insulin. The patient is put on a restricted diet, usually consisting of about six meals a day that are low in starch but high in protein so as not to abnormally raise the blood sugar. It is an effective treatment. By regulating the sugar, we don't set the pancreas into a flurry of reaction. But I'll repeat again—this is a rare condition. Which is not to say that sugar is marvelous for you.

The "Sugar Blues" Phenomenon

Although they are not hypoglycemic, there are a number of patients who have come into my office willing to swear that sugar and sweets are affecting their moods. It would be easy to dismiss this as pure hypochondria. I am not an adherent of the "sugar blues" philosophy. But I have heard this complaint often enough that I am willing to allow some basis to it.

As we have noted, there seems to be a tenuous connection between blood-sugar levels and a person's outlook. Elevated sugar makes some people anxious; lowering of the sugar seems to mildly depress people. Conversely, it has been noted that many depressed patients have blood-sugar levels that are somewhat on the high side (but then depression and anxiety are not mutually exclusive, so that's not as paradoxical as it might appear on the face of it). And what about the drug addicts with a craving for sweets, or the alcoholic who constantly wants candy? Can we be certain that there is not some hidden connection between glucose levels and what goes on in our mental functions?

I for one am not willing to swear to that. I believe these patients are not just imagining things, although where or what the connection might be is presently beyond the bounds of our knowledge. There might be some disturbance in insulin production, or there might be a malfunction in carbohydrate metabolism. As we have indicated in our discussion of hypoglycemia, paths do exist for altering our mood levels.

If you are a person who feels that sugar makes you moody, I would simply suggest that you try cutting your glucose intake. See if that makes you feel any better. At any rate, less sugar is not likely to hurt you.

The Chocolate Connection

Sugar is one thing; chocolate is another. There is a large amount of evidence that chocolate can disturb people. Chocolate often shows up in the diets of migraine sufferers, and I have had a number of depressed patients who have indulged in great chocolate binges.

Chocolate contains a rather obscure transmitter with the imposing name of *phenylethylamine*. To date it has not been very well studied, and there are few conclusions that can safely be drawn about it. But you will note that on the list of dietary taboos distributed to patients on MAO inhibitors, chocolate is the only sweet included, and it is because of this mood changer called phenylethylamine.

We believe that this chemical is an antidepressant. It may also

181

play a role in schizophrenia. There is some evidence, by no means conclusive yet, that it may exacerbate certain psychotic states. This may also explain why people who are depressed will sometimes find themselves attracted to chocolate. In their search to find pleasure, or to fill up the "empty space," they may be additionally gratified by the ingestion of this mood changer.

Food Additives and Hyperactivity

As I think may have become apparent by now, diet is not the most promising research path. While no one denies that it can affect our emotions, it is rarely the cause of the more deleterious mood disorders. There are reasons for this. We are complex organisms; every tissue, every cell is a miniature chemical plant. And as if nature knew what fools we are, we are reasonably well protected from the substances we put into ourselves.

Nevertheless, because foods are visible and because our internal chemistry remains hidden in obscurity, there is a natural tendency to become concerned and even frightened about the potential dangers of our "civilized" regimen. A perfect example of this is "junk food." The name itself implies our prejudice against it. To some extent it is a well-founded prejudice, because common sense tells us that this food lacks quality.

Nevertheless, many serious nutritionists will argue that "junk food" is an improper label. They point out, quite correctly, that it does have nutritional value and that, when metabolized, its ingredients are good for us. The problem is one of degree, not kind. Most "junk food" items are high in calories. They tend to load us with carbohydrates but are rather weak in the other nutrients.

Then there is the problem of food dyes and additives. We see these as another evil of modern society. Manufacturers add these "poisons" for shelf life and eye appeal, and our youngsters gobble them in prodigious quantities. Almost everything we eat has additives and coloring—our vegetables, our meats, our frozen-food products, even such "good" things as fruit juice and breakfast cereal, not to mention such horrors as candy and soda pop.

Our instincts may tell us that these chemicals must be bad for us, but our instincts may not be related to fact. It remains for science, slow and ponderous, to separate truth from emotionalism and prejudice.

Nowhere has this been better exemplified than in the modern research into *hyperactivity,* that strange and ill-defined condition that has created such controversy in our communities' school systems. Hyperactivity is a behavioral problem, usually coupled with a learning impairment, that seems to prevail among pre-pubescent boys and is frequently treated with stimulants like Ritalin. We really don't know too much about it except that it is a complaint among teachers and parents, and since it can affect a child's electroencephalograph, it has unfortunately been referred to as *minimal brain dysfunction.*

From the beginning this illness has been clouded with controversy. In the first place, it was extremely hard to define. Where does being a "Tom Sawyer" leave off and being mentally or neurologically impaired take over? The problem was compounded by the employment of drug therapy. This was first done by a doctor named Charles Bradley, who in the early 1940s learned that certain stimulants had paradoxical effects on rambunctious youngsters. By the 1970s it had become a "war." The authors of a popular book called *The Myth of the Hyperactive Child* argued quite persuasively that Ritalin was being used as a sociopolitical weapon.

Enter a doctor named Benjamin Feingold, who was not only a pediatrician but also an allergist. In 1974 he published a hypothesis which continues to be a center of controversy.

The basis of Feingold's hypothesis is this: In 1951, having left the field of pediatrics, Feingold settled in northern California, where he began to study the effects of certain flea bites. From these studies he learned that the allergen in fleas was a low-molecular-weight chemical known as a *hapten.* When the hapten combined with a larger-weight protein, it stimulated the body's defenses and produced an allergic reaction. This led Feingold to

183

become interested in food additives, since food additives are also low-molecular-weight compounds. He noted the similarities between food additives and aspirin, which has long been known to create intolerance among some people.

In 1965, while treating a woman for hives, Feingold stumbled across a strange coincidence. He prescribed a diet that was made up of items containing no preservatives, food dyes or salicylates. Some ten days later he got an unusual call from the patient's psychiatrist. "What did you do with that patient?" asked the psychiatrist. Feingold's additive-free diet had seemed to eliminate her aggressiveness!

Feingold widened his researches to the study of hyperactivity. He began prescribing his diet to hyperactive children. Their parents concocted the most painstaking menus, including home-made ice cream with no artificial colorings. The results of this experiment were genuinely astounding, showing an improvement rate of about 70 percent! Even the children's teachers were impressed—this diet had worked wonders on the kids' personalities.

But the saga wasn't over. The teachers were impressed, but clinical researchers were much more skeptical. In order for Feingold to be proven correct, his diet would have to withstand the most rigorous empiricism. The best validation of any theory is the "double blind" study, in which none of the participants knows what is really being scrutinized. Could Feingold's diet survive a battery of tests in which all emotionalism was totally eliminated?

The researchers faced some imposing problems. How could they apply the double-blind technique to the problem of food additives? How could they radically change a child's diet without either the child or his parents being aware of what was happening? And how could they objectively judge the improvement? Could they rely on the parents for this, who have such obvious involvement? Above all, how could they eliminate bias—the natural prejudice that exists toward food additives?

The initial studies were not very encouraging. One was conducted at the University of Pittsburgh, another at the University of Wisconsin, but neither validated Feingold's hypothesis. A further study in California switched natural cranberry juice with juice containing food dyes. Only 1 of the 22 children involved showed any significant worsening of behavior.

The Feingold hypothesis was all but destroyed, seeming to be just another blind alley in the history of medicine. There were pediatricians who still believed in it, but it was research that counted, and research was scoffing at it.

Then two Canadians, James Swanson and Marcel Kinsbourne, began to notice something unusual in their work with rats at the University of Toronto. They were studying the effects of additives on the activities of the brain cells, and had been giving the rats Red Dye Number 3, a chemical compound by the name of erythrosin. They noticed that this dye produced marked changes in the activity of both norepinephrine and dopamine neurotransmitters, but they didn't see any behavioral changes. Could it be that the dosages were insufficient? What if they significantly increased the quantity? Could this be the link that Feingold had been looking for?

Swanson and Kinsbourne devised a new test, which was procedurally different from previous studies. They took twenty hyperactive children and put them on a five-day additive-free diet. They made no attempt to conceal the diet, and they didn't rely on the opinions of parents. For control they took twenty normal children and put them through the exact same regimen. Then, after five days, they began giving "medicines." These were in the form of ordinary capsules. Some of the capsules were placebo, but there were others that contained a high dose of food additives.

Then they put all forty children through a little game of learning. The children were asked to take numbered animals and match them up with their appropriate zoo numbers. The control group children performed this beautifully. Their abilities showed virtually no change at all. But the hyperactive group, after swallowing the additives, showed a marked decline in their overall performance!

All this was reported in the *New York Times Magazine* of August 24, 1980, under the headline: NEW HOPE FOR HYPERACTIVE CHILDREN. It quoted a pediatrician from Tufts as saying that it definitely proved Dr. Feingold's hypothesis. Then about six weeks later, buried in the same magazine's "Letters to the Editor" column, the following letter by Dr. Alan Zametkin of the National Institute of Mental Health appeared:

> In spite of some excellent commentary, your article is misleading in several ways.
>
> The *Science* report by Kinsbourne and Swanson actually showed differences between normal and hyperactive groups on placebo, not on drug. The dose of additive they used may be way above what any child actually does ingest. There are no adequate intake data on what additives actually cross the brain. . . .
>
> The hard facts are that the more closely the Feingold diet was tested, the less it seemed there was to it.

And on the heels of that was another letter—this one from a mother in Englewood, New Jersey—saying that she had tried the diet on her hyperactive daughter, and the results were nothing less than miraculous!

What are we to make of all these contradictory statements? Should we go with the parents, or should we go with the clinicians? Should we completely disrupt the entire processed-food industry, or should we dismiss the issue as alarmist propaganda? Perhaps we can at least form a commonsense conclusion if we remember that science is extraordinarily cautious. What works individually will be viewed as a fluke until it is established statistically that it will work in all cases.

My experience as a scientist makes me question this diet, as it smacks so much of wishful thinking. On the other hand, my experience as a doctor says that it is probably foolish to ignore children's parents. Perhaps it would help to keep two things in mind: First, this diet is extremely demanding. To eliminate everything that is questionable in food requires the patience of a saint and much sacrifice from family members. Second, there have been studies that show that *parents* contribute to hyperactivity. Indeed, the most successful therapy for eliminating this problem has sometimes been aimed at the parents' own discipline habits. It has been suggested that the Feingold diet may be most effective because it changes home life. It gives the child a feeling that he is important, which in the long run may be the most valuable healing agent.

Tryptophan: The "Natural" Sleeping Pill

Earlier in this book, when I talked about depression, I mentioned a dietary substance called *tryptophan*. I said that there was evidence that it might help depression, and particularly that it might help some depressed people sleep better. When I am confronted by friends who say, "You're a psychiatrist—what can I take to get to sleep at night?," since it would be dangerous and foolish to write them a prescription, I often advise them to buy some tryptophan.

Tryptophan is a perfectly natural substance. It is found throughout the animal and plant kingdoms. It is also found in the human body, which, as a matter of fact, is how we first learned about it.

For more than a century it has been recognized by researchers that the human blood contains a vasoconstrictor; that is, there is an agent contained in the serum which shrinks, or constricts, our arteries and blood vessels. For many years this was considered a nuisance, because it made blood so difficult to work with. In 1948 scientists finally isolated this agent and gave it the name *serotonin*.

A year later a doctor named M.M. Rapport found that the chemical structure of serotonin was actually *5-hydroxytryptamine* —which, as it turned out later, is synthesized from food we eat. The substance in the food is a chemical called tryptophan. Our bodies are made up of a number of amino acids, of which tryptophan is only one. These amino acids are linked together into larger building blocks called proteins. Tryptophan is the amino acid that goes into the synthesis of serotonin. Since it is contained in virtually everything proteinous, there is no reason to think that any of us is deficient in it.

Nevertheless, we have reason to suspect that a dose of

tryptophan can be therapeutic. There is some slight evidence that it may help depression and a bit more evidence that it can relieve some insomnias. And the beautiful thing about it is that you don't need a prescription. It is available in any health-food store or drugstore. It is virtually harmless and nonaddictive, and you don't have to worry about accidental overdose.

Most insomnia is self-curing by nature. If we don't sleep one night, we'll sleep the next, and even if we don't sleep for several nights running, eventually we will, and we'll feel refreshed again. People tend to worry too much about sleep. They have it in their minds that they need a certain number of hours a night. In reality there is no norm when it comes to sleeping patterns—many people thrive on only a few hours of unconsciousness.

Despite all this, many insomniacs get worried. They are convinced that they are suffering and will be unable to function. And when worry isn't the problem, it's usually boredom. What is there to do when everyone else you know is sleeping?

Insomnia, I believe, is one of the greatest contributors to drug abuse and alcoholism. People try to knock themselves out, and after a while they become dependent on the substances they use to do this. We have already noted the perils of prolonged use of tranquilizers—they diminish in effectiveness until they are nothing but placebos—placebos that are worthless in terms of sedation yet still have the power to make people dependent upon them. Far worse than tranquilizers is the problem of alcohol, the abuse of which is our number-one drug problem. As a psychiatrist, I can't tell you the patients I have whose lives have been wrecked because they habitually drink too much. The insidiousness of alcohol is that it is high on the dependency scale with addiction only coming after longterm use. Because people notice no physical symptoms, they feel relatively safe in continuing their indulgence.

If I had a loved one who was having trouble sleeping, my first suggestion would be nonmedical therapy. There are many programs and sleeping aids available, from autohypnosis to machines that produce surflike noises. If these don't work, I'd suggest some tryptophan. It is the only substance I can endorse with impunity. Last on my list would be tranquilizers and sedatives—and I would *never* recommend either a barbiturate or alcohol.

Diet Pills and Acute Psychosis

In the middle of the research that went into this chapter, I got an emergency phone call from a frantic mother. Her daughter was acting acutely psychotic, rambling incoherently and behaving like an animal. Knowing the patient's history, I called the hospital and arranged for a bed. "You've got a patient coming in who I think is on diet pills. Make sure you search her as soon as she arrives. I have a suspicion she might try to smuggle some in with her."

Diet pills are an abomination. They have no place in a legitimate weight program. The good diet doctors do not prescribe them, and you will not find them sanctioned by an organization like Weight Watchers. But since we are talking here about diet and mental outlook, I would be remiss if I ignored these substances. Too many people who are in other ways health conscious have landed in the hospital through the use of these mood changers.

The patient I mentioned is a perfect example. I think her history might be illuminating. I have changed her name and a few of the particulars, but the pattern she describes is almost a classic one.

Evelyn is in her early twenties. She is the type of young woman many people would call emotional. She has been in my care for a number of years, and I have seen her through a number of difficulties. Regardless of Evelyn's personality problems, one of her hang-ups is that she thinks she is homely. She is not homely; in fact, she is pretty, but she tends to be a bit on the heavy side. This has become a consuming passion with her. Weight has become her personal *bête noire*. Whatever is wrong or lacking in her life, she is convinced that it can all be attributed to her heaviness.

The problem from a psychiatrist's viewpoint is that this obsession with skinniness causes undue emotional stress. We see it in illnesses like anorexia nervosa, and we see it with people who fall prey to diet quacks. Evelyn's problem became compounded dramatically because her father is a leading New York City pharmacist, which means that anything she wanted—including diet pills—could be easily obtained by some appropriate arm-twisting.

It may seem strange to a person on the outside that a doctor or a pharmacist could be so foolish. There are many stories about addiction in doctors' families, and the common reaction to them is, "*Them*, of all people! We thought they'd know better!" Well, let me point out that "experts" are human, and they are prey to the same social and familial pressures as anyone else. There are doctors, pharmacists and executives of drug companies who will do in private what they know to be foolhardy.

I assume it was the same situation with this pharmacist. I can imagine the scenes that took place at the dinner table: his daughter threatening, cajoling, tyrannizing, accusing him of being unloving and heartless toward her. So the man gave in. I had warned him not to, and I presume that professionally he knew that he shouldn't, but perhaps out of love, or pity—or hostility—he succumbed and brought home a bottle of diet pills.

What are these pills? They are basically amphetamines—even those that can be purchased by mail order and over-the-counter. Some are quite mild and so avoid the drug laws, but they all have an effect on one's neurotransmitter system. They release large amounts of catecholemine into the synapse. The catecholemine system consists of norepinephrine—and dopamine. The increased stimulation by norepinephrine and dopamine can lead to elevated blood pressure, agitation, or, in the case of Evelyn, a psychotic state.

The tragedy inherent in the prescription of diet pills is that the people who use them are frequently unstable. They think that weight is the cause of their unhappiness, when actually it is a symptom of a more basic problem. The real problem is often depression, and depression, as you know, can also mean mania. Diet pills can increase this mania, propelling the user toward the psychotic borderline. Once there, the ordeal may be only beginning. If the pills are discontinued, one's spirits will plummet, and this can lead to severe depression—and a need to eat to fill up the "empty spot."

So whatever you do, please don't use diet pills.

11

The Search for Ultimate Causes

Five or ten years ago the information discussed up to this point in the book would have given a reasonably coherent picture of modern psychiatry and the neurotransmitter hypothesis. But you will recall that in our preliminary discussion of this subject, I mentioned that science has a way of pulling surprises on us—it does not evolve in a logical progression but by fits and starts, full of pitfalls and stumbling blocks. We have come up against a nest of complexities. Having been so optimistic just a couple of years ago, we have since grown increasingly aware of the obstacles confronting us.

I suspect that if you asked the average psychiatrist today about her understanding of the state of psychochemistry, she would probably tell you that we have found the key, and the name of that key is neurotransmitters. I myself would have said the same thing not too long ago, since the transmitter theory has been so beguiling. But the events that have transpired in the past several years show that, if anything, we have barely scratched the surface.

If I were an artist and could put this diagrammatically, I would draw a picture that had three distinct levels. The first level would be the level of behavior—the outward signs of our abnormalities. This is the level on which Freud was operating and which preoccupied Kraepelin and the taxonomists. This level is so complex, so full of nuances, that it took several thousand years to come to grips with it.

But eventually it became apparent that this was just the surface, the epidermis that covered the monstrosity. As distorted, complex and confusing as it appeared, the first level did not really go to the heart of the problem. Then came reserpine and the neurotransmitter theory, and scientists took their first steps into the underground root system. "Here," we said, "we will find the answers, buried in these neuronal activities." I myself was a full-fledged believer, and my work contributed to the "monoamine hypothesis." I was fairly convinced that both depression and psychosis were linked to the activity of these neuronal tennis balls.

But now it is becoming clear that while neurotransmitters may be significant, there is yet a deeper level to which we have not descended. We catch glimpses of it—murky and mysterious—but the sense of its presence is becoming more and more palpable. The neurotransmitters are the paths we are following. They are the wires we are tracing in a faulty transmission. But it is becoming more and more evident that the heart of the problem may lie in whatever those wires are ultimately connected to.

Our drug research first led us to the discovery of transmitters, and it is drugs that are now leading us beyond our hypotheses into a world full of baffling complexities and paradoxes. For even as I write this, and even as you read it, there is a new crop of drugs hitting the test market. And this new generation is busily destroying many of our most cherished hypotheses.

A New Look at Depression

You will recall that, while talking about the causes of depression, we pinned most of our hopes on a rather simple conjecture: that if the transmitters were depleted, one's mood went down, but if they were restored, one was likely to feel more ebullient again. We centered our theories around two transmitter families—serotonin and norepinephrine. Either or both seemed equally implicated, since these were the transmitters the current drugs acted upon. These theories grew out of the observation that reserpine produced the same symptoms as depression. Since reserpine depleted these particular transmitters, we naturally assumed that we had discovered the mechanism.

But notice all the loopholes and paradoxes. Amphetamines also affected these transmitters, but, at least as applied to the majority of cases, they were not very successful in making patients feel better. We have also noted that antidepressants have occasionally been known to alleviate anxiety—but that doesn't jibe with the premise that increasing these transmitter levels will heighten emotionalism. And what are we to make of substances like tryptophan? Tryptophan is a precursor of serotonin. Why have we been unable to prove definitely that introducing tryptophan will alleviate despondency?

Obviously we have left many riddles unanswered, and often we have preferred to avert our gaze from them. We have no idea why lithium works or why some depressed people fail to respond to anything. Or what about this one: If depression is triggered by the depletion or lack of certain neurotransmitters, why have we not been able to discover this lack in either man or animals suffering from depressive symptoms? And why do the drugs take so long to act? Their affect on transmitters is almost immediate; so why does it inevitably take ten days or more before the patient shows any demonstrable behavior change?

We are beginning to suspect that there is but one explanation: The transmitter theory is an inadequate hypothesis. There is something missing—some clue, some breakthrough—that must be found before the picture will be clear to us. More likely, in fact, there are many missing pieces. There are so many areas that have not been explored yet. The answer may lie in yet another transmitter family or in some function or entity that is so far unknown to us.

There is a distinction in medicine between pathways and

causes. The former we refer to as *pathogenesis*. This is the route, or chain of events, that leads to the outbreak of identified symptoms. The latter is what we call *etiology*. *Etiology* means "source," or "origin." There are many illnesses for which we know the pathways but are still uncertain about the causes. Take a common illness like pneumonia, for instance. Pneumonia is caused by a bacterium or virus. Its pathogenesis is an increased white blood count, elevated temperature and fluid in the bronchial tubes. Traditionally, whenever we treated pneumonia, we could only attack the pathogenesis. We could lower the fever and try to facilitate breathing, but the rest was left to the body's defense mechanisms. In the majority of cases this usually worked well. Pneumonia is no longer a leading killer. But science had no delusions that ice packs and croup tents had any direct bearing upon the initial infection process.

The same mode of thought applies to a disease like depression. We have found a way to control and sometimes conquer it. But the more we learn about it, the more obvious our ignorance has become, until now even our initial premises look increasingly shaky to us.

Why this uncertainty? Because we have discovered new drugs that are muddying the waters. Not only are they different from the current antidepressants, some of them even work through seemingly opposite mechanisms!

In a later chapter, when I'm talking about drug lag, I'm going to express my opinion about FDA policies. There is a conservatism afoot that I feel is not only hurting Americans but is having a chaotic effect on the worldwide drug market. The only reason I'm mentioning it now is that it is important to realize for the next few pages that the drugs that I'm describing are not really new, they are only new to the US readership.

America, which has always considered itself modern and well within the vanguard of medical advancement, is actually, in terms of psychopharmacology, among the most backward and primitive of the industrialized societies. The drugs that we are using are twenty years old. To lay people they still seem new and revolutionary, but to a doctor in England, France or Japan the medicines we have been talking about are ancient history.

194

By the time this book has reached your hands, there may be ads in journals for a "new" antidepressant. It belongs to a family called *tetracyclics,* and it will be touted as being superior to tricyclics. Tetracyclics may be followed by other drugs. All these "new" drugs are simply imports from Europe. They have been used by a generation of doctors abroad, but the FDA has been slow in recognizing them.

The superiority of these new antidepressants has yet to be proved on a wide-scale basis. Indeed, until they are used in America, their long-range virtues will probably remain shadowy. But what is striking about them is their mode of action and the effects they are having on scientific theory. For whether or not they are actually better than the old drugs, they are opening up brand new channels of inquiry along several lines.

First, there is the line of *increased specificity.* Rather than affecting several transmitter families, some of these drugs attack much more selectively. Tricyclics, you remember, inhibit the uptake of both serotonin and norepinephrine. But there is a new tetracyclic by the name of *maprotiline,* which seems only to affect the norepinephrine reuptake process. Similarly there are other new drugs—they go by such names as *fluoxetine* and *zimelidine*—whose primary effect is on serotonin and which have negligible effects on the norepinephrine family.

The importance of this should be obvious. It gives us controls by which to measure our research. By knowing exactly which transmitter we are affecting, we may gain a truer picture of depression's real pathogenesis.

Scientists are pursuing a similar line with the other antidepressants, the MAO inhibitors. These drugs, you will recall, work by inhibiting the enzyme that destroys or metabolizes certain transmitter families. But now we know that there are *two* kinds of enzymes—MAO-A and MAO-B—and there are drugs that work exclusively on each, which we hope may eliminate some of the uglier side effects. MAO-A destroys serotonin and norepinephrine, but it has no effect on phenylethylamine. Phenylethylamine is the active ingredient that makes chocolate a forbidden food when an inhibitor has been prescribed. MAO-B destroys phenylethylamine, but does not effect norepinephrine or serotonin. Both of these enzymes still destroy tyramine, but if we can destroy that by other means, these inhibitors will be even safer for us.

Another fascinating drug is *mianserin*. This antidepressant throws all our previous theories into chaos. Rather than increasing our neurotransmitter levels, it has little or no effect on norepinephrine or serotonin! If mianserin turns out to be a good antidepressant, then all of our old hypotheses will be obsolescent. The raising or lowering of neurotransmitters will be viewed as secondary to the true cause of depression.

What, then, might the true cause be? Surely we have not just been dealing with coincidence. These transmitter levels must have to do with *something,* and that something must be relevant to our depressive mood disorders. Here we can only hazard some conjectures, which in turn are predicated upon two possibilities: Either we have been looking at the wrong neurotransmitters, or else we have misinterpreted what transmitters really do to us.

The first possibility has been given some credence lately by some research being done on the transmitter family called *histamines,* which played such a key role in our original drug discoveries. Histamines exist in many places in the body, and we are now reasonably sure that the brain is one of them. There is recent evidence that *all* antidepressants are powerful antagonists of histamine neuronal activity. The significance of this finding is still not clear, since other drugs are also antagonists to histamines. Therefore, it is doubtful that, wherever this path of thought leads us, histamines will emerge as the exclusive mechanism. Rather, what we suspect is that there is a complex of mechanisms, each in turn leading to other mechanisms, and so on and on throughout the skein of our nerve fibers, until something somewhere pushes the depression button.

The other possibility is that we have failed to decipher the true significance of our altered transmitter activity—that it is neither their depletion nor replenishment that affects us so much as it is the reaction of our receptor sites. You recall what we said about tardive dyskenesia—that it could be the result of hypersensitized receptor areas. We conjectured that as the transmitters were

196

depleted, new receptors sprung up to atone for the deficiency. If I can go back to our original comparison with a tennis game, let's suppose for a moment that our nerve connections are tennis courts. The players are the receptors, the net is the synapse, and the tennis balls being volleyed are the neurotransmitters.

Regulating this activity is an enzyme called a *modulator*. Through a metabolic process, it controls the number of volleys. Thus the ultimate goal is neither victory nor defeat, but a constant exchange of transmitters across the netline.

Now suppose something is introduced that causes a shortage of transmitters. The villain might be an illness, or it might be some drug. In either case there are now fewer tennis balls, and this will result in a slowdown of activity.

One way nature might counteract this obstacle is by instructing the players to exert themselves more. Each receptor might become more sensitive, volleying the transmitters with greater efficiency. If this is not sufficient, another recourse would be to add new receptors on the postsynaptic-nerve endings, This would have the effect of turning singles matches into doubles matches, the additional players increasing the efficiency ratio.

But now let's say that some other villain (which again might be an illness or some psychotropic substance) began throwing out new neurotransmitters, which flew in volleys toward the multiplied receptor sites. Now the activity would increase to a frenzy. Instead of a modulated volley, there would be uncontrolled chaos. Nature, in an attempt to keep the rhythm constant, might begin eliminating players to cut down the exchange activity.

Notice that there are a number of phenomena in play here. There is the quantity of transmitters, and there is the quantity of receptor sites. There is also an important enzyme, the modulator, whose role we will examine more closely in a minute. The disruptive force might be any outside agent with the power to increase or deplete the transmitter populace. This would create another variable—namely, an increase or decrease in the number of receptor sites.

What science is proposing—and this is only a hypothesis—is that it is not simply the number of transmitters that affects us, but the overall activity, the speed of the volley, after nature has made the receptor changes. This casts the picture into an entirely different perspective. It means that our emotions are conditional upon receptor sensitivity. More transmitters mean *decreased* sensitivity—and this could be how antidepressants work.

What a lot of researchers find comfortable in this hypothesis is that it might help explain "delayed onset of action." This is that mysterious period of time between the change in the transmitter levels and the lifting of the depression symptoms. If our emotions are conditional upon the adjustment of the receptor sites, then obviously it would take time for the drug to work—the time between the addition or subtraction of tennis balls and the countervailing subtraction or addition of playing partners.

But there is yet another suspect that must not be ignored; that obscure little fellow we call the modulator. It is this enzyme that is in charge of the rate of activity, and if it is deficient or absent, there is bound to be chaos.

One modulator that we have begun to pay attention to is an enzyme by the name of *tyrosine hydroxylase*. It seems to be pivotal in determining the rates of formation of certain transmitters like norepinephrine. In at least one recent study using desmethylimipramine, the generic name for Norpramin and Pertofran, it was found that after seven days on this tricyclic compound, there was a 30 percent decrease in tyrosine hydroxylase. This means that some drugs can also affect modulators. They are striking at the root of the whole control system. With a defect in modulators there is more random firing, and this might lead to eventual behavior change.

The picture that emerges, while intricate in its parts, can actually be stated in rather simple terms: Depression may be caused by the inability of neurons to contain their function within proper limitations. The antidepressants, whatever the variables, seem to dispel such chaos and reinstill discipline. They do this, presumably, for a long enough period to allow the patient's adaptive processes to readjust.

So much for revising the neurotransmitter theory. Obviously we

198

are still quite far from etiology. Because what made the neurons begin running amok? What caused the original change in the transmitter populace?

In our chapter on depression we cited two factors that seemed to play a role in triggering this illness. One was environment, or how the world affects us, and the other was genetics, our inherited programming. We have no big breakthroughs in either of these areas—only the James-Lange theory (see p. 59) and the tenuous X-chromosome hypothesis (see pp. 99–100). Both of these are highly speculative, simply direction indicators for future research. The one thing we can say with reasonable assuredness is that when we arrive at the cause, it will probably be multiple. It is doubtful that there is any single villain that is solely responsible for this unpleasant affective disorder. We can presume that there is an inherited factor in some people that may predispose them to the onset of symptoms. We might also assume that few of us are immune if the disappointments in life are severe and traumatic enough. What we are doing now is threading our way through the sequences. We are a little like fishermen trying to sort out a backlash. Eventually we will find the original snag, and the beacon that guides us to it will probably be chemical.

Meanwhile, as doctors, we have a transcendent duty to improve diagnostic and therapeutic techniques. Simply because the etiology is obscure does not mean that we must surrender to the illness. I have already mentioned that there are new kinds of drugs. You will find them listed on page 204. But there are a couple of other avenues that are being explored, and I would be remiss if I didn't at least mention them to you.

A couple of years ago, when our hypotheses were simpler, we felt certain that we had struck upon a new diagnostic tool. As it has turned out, there are a number of problems attached to it, but it may yet develop into something valuable. There is a substance in the body called *MHPG*. It's a metabolite, a waste product—3-methoxy-4-hydroxyphenylglycol. It is created by the destruction of norepinephrine, and thus might be used as a measurement of its precursor. Where MHPG abounds in the urine, it would seem to indicate high norepinephrine activity. Conversely, if you found a dearth of this substance, you might postulate a deficiency in the transmitter that it comes from.

Unfortunately, this theory has complications, and one of them is that levels of norepinephrine are not a measurement of depression symptoms. Antidepressants may increase norepinephrine, but depression does not seem to indicate deficiency. As a consequence, we have not been able to judge a person's feelings simply by measuring MHPG in a urine sample.

However, MHPG might be a useful assaying agent. We can use it to determine the reaction caused by certain drugs; those that act upon norepinephrine will result in an increase of this stuff in the urine samples. Tofranil, for example, the brand name for imipramine, definitely increases norepinephrine, and there is some indication that it may be preferred for patients who have a low MHPG level. On the other hand, Elavil seems to increase serotonin and doesn't seem to do much for norepinephrine. So if a patient comes in showing high MHPG, we might presume that Elavil will have greater potency.

All of this may sound very intriguing but it does not suggest, as one author said recently, that doctors who practice psychopharmacology have replaced the couch with the urinanalysis bottle. In fact, we feel certain that this will never be possible. MHPG levels are very delicate. The regimen required to get an accurate reading is more than most patients are willing to put themselves through. For example, no drugs would be permitted for an extended period. This is all right if the patient is healthy, but if he is anxious and depressed it may be too much to ask. Bananas and all foods with norepinephrine are also taboo. The norepinephrine never reaches the brain cells, but it does show up in the urine, and there is no way of determining its point of origin. And vanilla isn't allowed because when it hits the stomach it is also metabolized into an MHPG substance, and that would show up in the urine samples—which, by the way, require an all-day bathroom process. So it is safe to assume that whatever the future holds, MHPG will require a lot more refinement—which is not to say that we won't someday be using it or that it will never have a place in day-to-day office practice.

While we're on the subject of interesting phenomena that have yet to find their place in the treatment of depression, one line of research that we may yet hear more about is an area of inquiry called *sleep-deprivation therapy*. Sleep has recently become a fascinating topic. Around the world there are teams of researchers studying various aspects of the layers of unconsciousness. Psychiatry is scrutinizing this subject quite closely. Sleep and dreams are so obviously relevant to us, and it is not without thought that we make comparisons between certain psychoses and the sensations of dream experiences.

As we noted quite prominently in our material on depression, the disruption of sleep patterns is a classic symptom of the disease. There seems to be some fundamental connection between depression and insomnia that makes the latter a necessary ingredient of the illness. But the truth is that we don't know much about it. We have only begun to fathom how sleep affects our transmitter mechanisms. We know that serotonin seems to be a helpful sleep inducer, but beyond that our knowledge is fragmentary.

Nevertheless, there have been some interesting findings that help dramatize the relevance of sleep to mood disorder, and one of them is that lack of sleep seems to have the short-term effect of *relieving* depressive states!

This, of course, is a very odd finding. Sleeplessness is a vegetative symptom of depression. And yet in some 25 percent of depressed patients studied, going without sleep seems to alleviate their symptoms.

We can only speculate on some of the reasons for this—we certainly don't know the chemical mechanisms—but it leads us to conclude that our popularly held conceptions are not consistent with emerging research findings. For example, most people will say that if they go without sleep one night, they will feel cranky and irritable the next day. They will blame this discomfort on their failure to sleep, perceiving insomnia to be the source of their edginess. This does not jibe with recent research. Insomnia and crankiness may be related, but the former is not the cause of the latter; rather, both are symptoms of some unknown disturbance somewhere.

How do we know this? If you have spent all your life sleeping from midnight till eight, and then suddenly you are asked to work the night shift, the change creates an extreme unpleasantness in your psychic outlook. It does not matter that you have slept during the day—you are still going to feel listless, lethargic and irritable. Factory hands, police officers and disc jockeys all know this, as does anyone who has ever suffered from "jet lag."

We can reproduce this phenomenon experimentally by having volunteers stay up all night. Then, when they are put to sleep for a solid eight hours, it will have no effect on their tiredness or edginess. This has led to the current perception that sleep is part of a rhythmic process, and that it is the rhythm that governs our emotional outlook and not the sleep itself, either in quantity or quality. It is true that sleep is a necessary activity, and so are the various stages that we go through in our sleep period. But insomnia per se is not the problem—the difficulty lies deeper, either neuronally or psychically.

This leads us to wonder if one of the symptoms of depression— insomnia, or disrupted sleep patterns—might not actually be a natural defense mechanism, an attempt to combat some deeper pathology. In other words, when you can't sleep at night and the following day you have a hard time concentrating, your sleeplessness may be your body's way of trying to deal with whatever is troubling you. Many depressed patients are convinced that insomnia is the cause of their discomfort. But when they are forced to stay up, to keep going all night, they will actually perform better on the tasks that are assigned to them.

Unfortunately, in terms of realistic therapy, sleep deprivation is not very practical. You can't force a patient to stay up all the time so that, though she is exhausted, she will have a rosier outlook. What we may ask of a patient is that she try it sporadically. Often we will try it in conjunction with drug therapy. While sleeplessness itself is only a temporary remedy, it can have short-term effects on a patient's outlook.

More to the point is what all this may mean to research. Is circadian rhythm a factor in depression? And if so, how? What is its mechanism? How do such diurnal forces play a role in our thought processes? There may be some antidepressant, endogenous in origin, that is released in our brains after sleep is denied us. But if so, what is it? Where does it come from? Can we reproduce it for use as a future drug treatment?

The answers to these questions lie buried in the future. I would think that by 1990 we will probably know a lot of them, meaning that the *third* generation of antidepressants will be far superior to anything now available. In the meantime one of the results of these studies is to drive another nail into the coffin of sleeping pills as treatment. It is becoming increasingly clear that the risks of taking them far outweigh the alleged benefits. We see this in more and more hospitals, as patients are no longer awakened to take a sedative. We are beginning to realize that, whatever sleep does for us, it is but one integral part of a much larger bio-picture.

Deeper into Schizophrenia

If you've followed me this far, you may have noticed the similarity between our theories about depression and schizophrenia. Both are pegged to a view of transmitter activities, and both arose from some elementary drug experiments. In the case of depression it was the "reserpine syndrome," and in the case of schizophrenia it was the effect of amphetamines on rat behavior. Unfortunately, as depression is proving somewhat more complicated, so our views on schizophrenia have also been challenged.

Schizophrenia, you'll recall, fit the simple hypothesis that the psychosis is linked to dopamine-transmitter levels. Introduce drugs that reduce those levels and you will eliminate many of the psychotic features. No one is prepared yet to discard that theory—there does seem to be a connection between schizophrenia and dopamine—but when we reexamine it in a brighter light, not all the pieces fit together quite comfortably.

For one thing, we have the problem of *onset of action*. Drugs

Some of the New Antidepressants
and How They Work

Name	Mechanism of Action	Hoped-for Benefit
maprotiline (trade name, Ludiomil)	selective norepine- phrine inhibitor; neg- ligible effect on serotonin	fewer anticholinergic effects; may be faster acting for some pa- tients
fluoxetine	selective serotonin inhibitor	efficacy not clear yet
zimelidine	selective serotonin inhibitor	efficacy not clear yet
trazodone	inhibits serotonin cen- trally but increases it peripherally	appears to have fewer side effects and may be faster acting
mianserin	no effect on uptake of norepinephrine, dopamine or serotonin	few side effects and more rapid action

work to block dopamine almost immediately. Yet often it will take several days or even weeks before we see anything resembling therapeutic activity.

Another conundrum: When we give L-Dopa, a building block or loader of the dopamine transmitter, to a patient along with antipsychotics, we will sometimes see an additional improvement. It has also been noted that while L-Dopa alone seems to increase or exacerbate many symptoms of psychosis, it sometimes has no effect on focal symptoms such as hallucinations and logical-thought disorder.

So what are we to make of these contradictions? Should we just throw up our hands and say, "It's the work of the devil"? Absolutely not—and I'm going to try to explain why, because it is essential to an understanding of medicine.

Science moves forward on the back of error. If it weren't for error, there would be no progress. Hypotheses are goals. They are approximations. In some ways they are fantasies of what awaits us at the end of the rainbow. They goad us forward; they lose their attractiveness, we form better hypotheses and we all march forward again. For the past twenty years the transmitter hypothesis has been the guiding star that we have set our sights on. It has led us to some of the most astounding discoveries in the history of medicine and total revolution in the field of psychiatry. Now that we are closer we see that our goddess has warts. She is not quite the beauty that we originally envisioned. Yet any hypothesis that can create such progress deserves a special shrine in the history of the sciences. Look back a minute to see the ground that has been covered. We have come from *The Snake Pit*, those gray sanitariums, and we have saved countless lives and untold suffering, and we have restored a measure of dignity to the world's largest leper colony, not to mention the knowledge we have gained. We have gone from the abstract guesswork of ego and libido into the darker reaches of neurology and chemistry, relieving more pain in a year than in all of previous history. It has truly been an inner-space program. The transmitter theory was our lunar landing. But now it is beginning to outlive its usefulness, and we want to move on toward the ultimate causes.

I have alluded to the fact that genetic predisposition plays an indisputable role in chronic schizophrenia. This truth alone has many implications with which we, as social beings, have yet to grapple. There is the question, for instance, of genetic counseling—how are we to tread the delicate path between the duty to inform and needless alarmism?

In a recent review for the National Institute of Mental Health, Dr. Seymour Kessler of the University of California pointed out some of the obstacles that will have to be overcome if we are to have constructive counseling programs. One problem, of course, is that lacking sound diagnostic weapons (such as the employment of amniocentesis, for instance), we find ourselves in the unenviable position of trying to make guesses on the basis of statistical tables. Statistics are useful—but how relevant are they to the patient? Suppose you wanted to know your chances of giving birth to a schizophrenic. If I told you your risk was one out of seven, would you and your spouse really know how to proceed on that? This problem is worsened by the nature of the illness. Our understanding of schizophrenia is burdened with fear and emotion; it carries a stigma of inadequacy and guilt not usually associated with Tay-Sachs disease or sickle-cell anemia.

While such counseling is available even now, we are far from satisfied by the quality or simplicity of it. We're going to have to dig deeper into the etiology of the disease to provide the public with the awareness that it deserves.

Later on we're going to look into the future and talk about the prospects of genetic engineering; for it is here that we must eventually focus our research if we are to be totally free of these mental pathologies. But, at least for now, in regard to schizophrenia, such speculations are in the realm of fantasy. For how can we know what we're even looking for when the parameters of the illness are still so murky to us?

Let us allow for the moment that the problem is genetic. That is not a very unreasonable assumption considering that there have been so many twin and adoption studies that support the Rosenthal-Kety findings discussed on pages 148–50. But where does this lead us? Is genetics the end? Should our investigation stop at the discovery of a little, malformed cell speck? Or are there other factors, still unknowable, that might play a role even in creating the mutation?

A few years ago Herbert Meltzer, a professor of psychiatry at the University of Chicago, came up with an interesting observation that is still lying on the back burners of psychiatric inquiry. There is an enzyme in our bodies, *creatine phosphokinase*, which researchers usually refer to as *CPK*. It catalyzes the reaction between two other substances to create two agents called *creatine* and *adenosine triphosphate*. It comes in three different forms in three different body parts—the brain, the heart and the skeletal muscle. The CPK in skeletal muscle cannot pass through the blood-brain barrier.

In working with a group of severe psychotics, Meltzer found a significant elevation of CPK in their blood. It was the type of CPK one finds in skeletal muscle and is usually associated with some sort of muscle damage. As he cast the net further, it became increasingly evident that the people who had this were not just schizophrenics—they included a wide variety of seriously ill patients, including manic-depressives and even some senile people. What did it mean? Meltzer wasn't sure. But other researchers began to replicate his findings. There was no doubt about it: People with severe psychosis had levels of CPK far in excess of normal people.

And here is something of even stranger import: When Meltzer tested these psychotics' relatives, he found that up to 40 percent of them had the same aberration—even those who had no mental problem!

If you think about this for a minute or two, a couple of possibilities begin to emerge: One is that creatine phosphokinase may be the predictive ingredient that science has been looking for. Remember the problems of genetic counseling—all we have to go on is statistical probabilities. What we need is some clue, some valid test that will pinpoint the risks for each individual. Might CPK prove to be that clue? So far, we don't know—our knowledge is still too primitive. But in years to come, when we find this elevated enzyme in someone, we might be able to target that person as being a high-risk psychosis carrier.

There is another avenue that is also enticing. I said that CPK is associated with muscle damage. So is psychosis. This is well established. We have noted numerous changes in the muscles of mental patients. An observation like this helps us make a leap in our thinking. Now we are talking about something biological. We are saying that there is a germ, a life form that is eating the muscle and creating abnormal quantities of this particular enzyme.

We are saying, quite simply, that it could be a virus.

This, of course, is highly speculative, but it falls within the boundaries of valid hypothesizing. At the end of the trail, when all is said and done, we may find that the culprit is a foreign organism. This virus might infect people through a number of pathways. Perhaps it is a virus that damages dopamine. Perhaps it is a virus so small, so subtle, that it plays havoc with our very gene structure. Notice the number of questions this might answer for us. Why does schizophrenia take so long to appear? Why is the illness chronic in some cases, while in others it comes and goes intermittently? We might be dealing with a very unusual little organism that takes months or years or even decades to incubate. Only when it reaches a certain development might it trigger the processes that result in psychosis.

Independent of Meltzer and his findings, there have been several studies that substantiate this viewpoint. One, for example, by a scientist named Pulkkinen, delves into the role played by *immunoglobulins*, which are a kind of blood protein that help transport various antibodies. Antibodies, of course, are natural defense substances, and being at either high or low levels may be the sign of an infection somewhere. Pulkkinen found that withdrawn patients showed unusually high levels of one kind of antibody, while paranoid patients, at the opposite end, seemed to be deficient in this same kind of protein substance. Pulkkinen suggested that the reason for this discrepancy might be that paranoid patients are more susceptible to stress. Generally, he noted, there was a correlation between higher antibody levels and shorter hospital stays.

In another study, done in 1978, investigators took spinal taps of various mental patients. They wanted to measure immunoglobulins and viral antibodies in the cerebrospinal fluid, or CSF, which surrounds the brain and spinal cord. It is generally considered the best means available of analyzing substances in contact with the brain area. They found that six out of seventeen patients with serious schizophrenia had elevations of the IgG antibody. What is odd about this is that the IgG antibody is the same antibody that opposes the measles virus!

On the heels of this, in 1979 came word from England that a group of researchers had identified an agent with certain viral properties in the spinal fluid of schizophreniform patients. Because they didn't know what to name it, they simply called it a *viruslike agent*. This has been shortened to VLA—a primitive label, but the best now available. VLA seems to damage human cells, particularly a cell from tissues of the lung. It was also shown that patients with this agent had elevated levels of a certain kind of antibody.

The significance of this will, I hope, be apparent. It is one thing when you are talking about genetics or dopamine: As far as genetics is concerned, our knowledge is inadequate, and in trying to understand dopamine we are mired in pathogenesis. A virus, however, presents a whole new ball game. *If we can find a virus, we can find a vaccine*. Is it remotely possible that within the next twenty years we will have banished schizophrenia as we have banished smallpox?

A breakthrough like that doesn't come along very often. But if it does, it is entirely possible that these findings will have laid the groundwork for it.

Wrapping up our discussion of this most dreadful of illnesses, it seems to come in a variety of forms. And each form, in turn, might have a variety of causes, at the far end of which might be several etiologies. There is a probable connection with dopamine activity, and there is statistical evidence of genetic predisposition. Finally, there is a glimmer of hope that at the end of our search, we will identify a virus. What you have read in this book is but an interim report. The final chapter will be written sometime in the future. But it is a story whose plot is thickening intriguingly—and, for the first time in history, there is the sense of an outcome.

Beyond Valium

In preparing this book, while talking to researchers, there was an almost universal reaction whenever the title was mentioned: "Why are you choosing to focus on Valium when it is the least important drug in the scientific scheme of things?" The answer, of course, is transparently simple: It is the drug most identified with psychiatric therapy; and it is also the symbol of a fascinating research effort, one whose benefits and risks seem to be intimately entwined. It is also not a trivial drug. Valium is a symbol of either hope or damnation for millions of people.

But if my sense is correct, there is an attitude among journalists that amounts to an ax being ground whenever Valium is derogated. And there is obviously no shortage of ammunition. We have seen that the overuse of Valium is to be avoided. It creates dependency, it creates addiction and, after a short period of use, it may not even do any good.

Nevertheless, as a practicing psychiatrist, I worry that in our zeal to protect some people from drug abuse we aren't damaging others who need tranquilizers desperately. I have had anxious and depressed people come into my office who, if I took away their tranquilizers, would be lost to all therapy. They might steal tranquilizers, or they might take to alcohol, or they might lose their jobs, their families, their dignity. It is the same dilemma we faced with alcohol during Prohibition. And alcohol abuse in America today is a far bigger problem than our dependence on tranquilizers.

So even if Valium has some imperfect aspects, its positive effects remain a worthy objective. We need to understand anxiety better, and we need a substance that will ameliorate its ravages.

As may be apparent from what you have read so far, Valium is different from either Thorazine or Tofranil: We have not sufficiently understood it to include it comfortably in the transmitter hypothesis. We know, of course, that it works on transmitters, but the principles of its action have remained blurred and hazy. And until we understand what it does in our bodies, there is little hope of finding a drug that will be better for us.

Yet finding such a drug has become an absolute imperative. Not only would it be welcome for therapeutic purposes, it would also be welcomed by those people whose business it is to make profits for stockholders. Let's not have any illusions about this. Drugs are business. They are important commerce. Few people can afford to ignore the lure of the profit motive. Pharmaceutical manufacturers are no exception. They live or die by their annual sales figures—and when you have a product that is as popular as Valium has been, there is a powerful motive to return to that well again.

Toward the end of this book I'm going to be talking about drug companies, and we'll examine the politics that go into their research. However, drug companies should not be made the scapegoats; scientists, too, play a very big role. But beyond the cynicism we can all apply to these matters, I sincerely believe that there is integrity in the drug industry. Admittedly, this integrity is often imposed by society, but I believe there is more of it than one might find in many other enterprises.

A product like Valium is a perfect example. If you have ever glanced through a medical journal, you saw that the ads touting the various products are of a different caliber than one finds in consumer advertising. There are no false claims. There is no hyperbole. Everything is spelled out as objectively as possible. In fact, sometimes the list of contraindications is longer and more detailed than the hoped-for benefits!

In the past couple of years, since Valium has been challenged, the ads for this product have acquired a new character. Very often on the opposing page there is a cautionary note that is downright startling. In big, bold type doctors will be warned against the dangers inherent in Valium dependency. They are also advised to scrutinize patients carefully, looking for the telltale signs of potential drug abusers.

It is easy to imagine some of the motives for this. First of all, there's the FDA, which applies such conservative standards that it's a challenge for a copywriter to say anything good about something. There is also the skepticism inherent in the audience. Doctors tend not to be turned on by hucksterism. Finally, one might suppose that with Valium sales waning, there might be a corporate mood of "we have nothing to lose" involved.

Nevertheless, it is an unusual spectacle, and one might wish for such honesty in other forms of advertising. Wouldn't it be instructive if automobile manufacturers listed all the defects one might encounter in their products?

Since drug manufacturing is so competitive, and minor tranquilizers account for so much profit, one can only speculate on the research activity presently being deployed to supercede Valium. During the preparation of this book, we invited representatives of several drug companies to share some clues as to where their research was taking them. They refused, naturally fearful lest something they told us might tip off their competitors. As a scientist, however, I can make an educated guess. There have been some significant new studies on tranquilizer mechanisms, and these, in turn, are opening new research paths that the major drug companies will be quick to scurry down.

When we talked about the benzodiazepines on page 42, I mentioned Lowell Randall, who was testing the effects of muscle relaxants. He did this by injecting drugs into lab mice and placing them on a screen that was tilted at an angle. Researchers no longer use this test. They use a chemical called *pentylenetetrazol*. It goes by the trade name of Metrazol, and when you inject it into a rat, it creates a muscle seizure.

Benzodiazepines—the "minor tranquilizers"—are selectively effective at preventing these seizures. This has led scientists to look for the mechanisms that are responsible for creating these Metrazol seizures.

During the course of this research in the past few years, interest has centered on a transmitter called *GABA* (gamma-aminobutyric acid). GABA is what is called an *inhibitory transmitter*. That is, it suppresses neuronal activity. It exists in the brain and in other nerve areas, and it seems to play a role in Metrazol muscle seizure.

When scientists began to experiment on GABA, they came across an interesting discovery: Valium seemed to have *two* effects on it, depending on where the GABA was located. In the spinal cord of a cat, for example, Valium potentiated GABA's inhibiting power. In other areas of the brain, however, Valium worked to reduce this same GABA effect.

How Valium did this was the next logical question, but here the researchers encountered a mystery. There was no evidence of increased release or that GABA was being blocked at reuptake. Since GABA is found at the presynaptic nerve ending, scientists began to suspect that they ought to look elsewhere. Perhaps they should go "across the channel" and see what was happening on the postsynaptic receptor side.

To take this journey they used radioactive Valium. This is Valium which has been treated so that its activities can be traced.

212

The scientists fully expected to find that Valium was binding at the GABA receptor stations.

And, indeed, they did find that Valium had binding sites. The sites were located in the mammalian brain, but they also found them in the kidney, the liver, the lung and various other parts of the anatomy. Eventually they found them in the human brain. Only when they found all these sites, they discovered that the sites at which the Valium was binding were not the same sites that were attracting the GABA compound! How could this be?

There is a phenomenon in our nerve cells in which receptor sites work in near proximity. They are close to each other, and they are very similar, only they work as a team, a kind of *molecular complex*. Valium seems to influence GABA. GABA, we know, has its own receptors. But next to these receptors, working in harmony, are other receptors with an affinity for Valium molecules.

This would indicate that, as well as GABA, there is some other substance that must bind like Valium does. Scientists began to look a bit closer. They ran some studies involving animal breeding. And what they found was very intriguing in light of what we commonly call personality differences.

You see, rats can be bred to have different personalities. They can be made ferocious, or meek, or extroverted. Their sex can also be predetermined, and a female can be made to have all the male sex habits. And one of the traits which can be bred into rats is the quality of bravery, courage or valor. Conversely, one can also breed timid rats—rats so scared that they will be frightened of everything.

What researchers have found is that timid or fearful rats have significantly fewer Valium receptor sites, and that rats that have been bred to be brave and more assertive have more sites that seem expressly tailored for tranquilizers!

And beyond that, it has also been found that when you subject a rat to a series of shock traumas, a substance like Valium will very quickly lose its ability to bind at the receptor areas!

What all this could mean in terms of future research is so fascinating that it may sound like science fiction. Are we to assume from this that drugs like Valium are a chemical key to bravery and heroism? Is there a built-in reason that some people need Valium? Do they need it to make up for a receptor deficiency? Is this why some people are so cool and unflappable, while others become unglued as soon as life throws a curve at them? And is this also what contributes to the "emotional breaking point"? If a series of traumas will deaden these receptors, then this might explain why even the toughest of heroes must eventually crack under torture or questioning. Is coolness inherited? Are there gender differences? The implications are sundry and titillating. But that is all they are, because there is nothing to substantiate them—it is just an interesting path that remains to be traveled someday.

Right now the search is on for "endogenous Valium"—a natural substance that can work like a tranquilizer. That search is more difficult than one might assume, because even when we find it, there are bound to be difficulties.

In a recent issue of *New York* magazine, there was a cover story called "Medicines for the Eighties." It was a pretty good roundup of a number of new substances, some of which bear on psychiatry. I was amused to note that one of these substances was an anxiolytic called *Gamma Compound.* It was touted to be a naturally produced Valium that some scientists had abstracted from a number of urine samples.

I assume that "Gamma Compound" is actually GABA. The prefix for GABA is the Greek word *gamma,* and I imagine that what got stuck in the typewriter was gamma-aminobutyric acid. Be that as it may, the gist of the article was that discovery of a "natural Valium" was just around the corner.

This may well be—but there are problems attached. The body is like a fortress, with an inside and an outside. It uses tissues, capillaries, membranes and enzymes to keep outside substances from invading its privacy. And it will do the same thing with a natural tranquilizer. There are enzymes and processes that will try to discourage it. You cannot simply swallow a pill made of GABA and think that it will get from your stomach to your brain cells.

So we are still some distance from a natural tranquilizer. Some precursor of GABA might be the solution. But there are other

214

solutions that are perhaps a bit more promising, particularly since GABA does not lock into Valium receptors.

Now that it is known that we have these receptors and we are beginning to discover their principles of action, two substances receiving a lot of attention are *purines* and a compound called *nicotinamide*. This latter, you will recall, is one of the elements that figured so heavily in the "transmethylation theory" (see p. 153). It was thought that giving it to schizophrenics would help neutralize their "endogenous hallucinogens." Now nicotinamide has popped up again, as a Valium mimic. It has been found that it binds to benzodiazepine receptors. It does not bind nearly so well as Valium, but that it does so at all is a promising research lead.

Purines, the end product of nucleoprotein digestion, first gained prominence in the 1940s, when it was found that some derivatives of them—"antipurines"—were useful in combatting leukemia. One antipurine called *6-mercaptopurine* is still being used against leukemia, and a derivative of this, *azathioprine*, is used to prevent the rejection of organ transplants.

Now we have learned that certain of these purine substances have a marked affinity for Valium receptor sites. We have also found an intestinal peptide whose attraction to these receptors is remarkably powerful.

There are some other tidbits that might prove useful. There is a substance, for example, called *triazolopyridazine*. It is of a totally different structure from Valium, yet its effects on animals seem to be quite similar. The remarkable thing about triazolopyridazine is that it doesn't become more dangerous when mixed with alcohol. This could be an important safety feature in a society where John Barleycorn is still so predominant.

If I were to hazard a guess, I would say that within the near future we will see a significant breakthrough toward finding a Valium successor. Until then, we must simply get along as best we can, exercising prudence and caution with a drug that has many drawbacks.

12

Placebo and Biofeedback—
The Mind as Healer

"When all is said and done," the medical director of a large pharmaceutical company was quoted as saying recently, "the best drug that psychiatrists have may yet turn out to be placebo."

I'll assume he was saying this with a bit of a twinkle; if not, his company is headed for trouble. Nevertheless, there was reason in his irony: Placebo is indeed an important medicine.

There is a wonderful story about how this word came to be a synonym for "make-believe medicine." It goes like this:

In the early years of this century when patent medicines were in vogue, certain legislators and medical experts decided to prove that these medicines were worthless. Congressional hearings were arranged under the leadership of a Senator Placebo. The Senator insisted that the hearings be closed to the public, but reporters' interviews with witnesses soon revealed that all expert testimony concluded that the patent medicines were indeed worthless. There began to be a hue and cry for a hearings report.

Finally Senator Placebo made his report:

"There will be no report," he said. "I have destroyed all records of the hearings. No medical evidence was given to prove that the medicines were in any way harmful. They are safe, so why should I deny their effect?" And ever after, drugs with no effects were called "placebos."

Of course there is no truth to this charming anecdote; the Senate has yet to see a "Placebo"; but the story does have sentimental veracity and, like Aesop's fables, it deserves reiterating. The more accepted etymology of this strange-sounding word is that it is the first-person singular of the Latin *placere,* meaning "to please." The word also appears in Psalm 116 (*Placebo Domino in regione vivorum,* "I will please the Lord in the land of the living"), which was sung at funerals.

The word has always had a hypocritical edge to it. Fake mourners were said to be "singing their placebos." Slowly through the centuries it crept into science, until by 1894 it meant "make-believe medicine."

This usage is presumptuous, when you come to think of it, because medicine through the ages was *all* placebo: the leeches, the compresses, the elixirs, the blood-letting—all were pretty useless in terms of biology. A colleague of mine, Dr. Arthur K. Shapiro, has written a monograph on the use of placebo. In it he includes a minicompendium of some of the "medicines" from bygone ages:

> crocodile dung, teeth of swine, hooves of asses, spermatic fluid of frogs, eunuch fat, fly specks, lozenges of dried vipers, powder of precious stones, bricks, fur, feathers, hair, human perspiration, oil of ants, earthworms, wolves, spiders, moss scraped from the skull of a victim of violent death . . .

And so on.

But here's the significance—a lot of these worked! Sick people took them and recovered. This went on for thousands of years, and the doctors who prescribed these medicines were treated as holy men.

In *Psychopharmacology: From Theory to Practice,* **Dr.** **Adolf** Pfefferbaum of Stanford University makes the quizzical comment that now that we have *real* medicine, doctors seem to have lost a lot of their esteem in society. This may be true. The magic is gone. People grumble about quacks and charlatans. As medicine has become more mechanistic, it has become fairer game for the skeptics and nay-sayers. Dr. William Nolen, in his best-seller *Healing,* showed how even sophisticates can still believe in magic. Look, he said, at how many people accepted *The Exorcist* as an authoritative document.

Healing through religion may be a powerful placebo. I have had a number of patients with whom therapy has failed, but what I couldn't accomplish a religion did—whether Christian, Jewish, Muslim or Hindu. I have sometimes been known to make eyebrows lift when I express my admiration for Oral Roberts. It's not that I share his beliefs or theology, but I recognize the efficacy of his way of doing things. I was fascinated to read that Oral Roberts University has been planning to build a giant new medical center which will have all the latest equipment and technology, but will also pay homage to things that are "spiritual." As I understand it, every patient in this hospital will be assigned an aide, called a Prayer Partner. Together, the patient and the specially trained Prayer Partner will join in expressing the ideals of their piety.

In big cities like New York, we are too worldly for that. If I were to suggest such a thing at my hospital's next staff meeting, there would be shocked stupefaction, probably followed by the opinion that poor old Rosenblatt is ready for retirement. But I have seen ample evidence that the mind can work wonders. There is more to medicine than the swallowing of a capsule. And although doctors may know this, we hate to discuss it, because to do so might erode our authority still further.

Today we depend on a new kind of cultism. Gone are the witch doctors, the feathers, the crocodile dung; and in their place we have chemical formulas, esoteric jargon and the rules of empiricism. All of these have their justification, but they also place authority in the hands of the healer. And it is this authority, this faith in the master, that invests us with much of our ability to heal people. It has been proven in study after study that those who believe have a tendency to recover; those who do not have a higher morbidity pattern. Yet scientifically, for the sake of empiricism, we judge all new drugs against a standard of skepticism. It is the disparity that exists between placebo and real drug that we use to measure the real drug's efficacy.

That is why when we are talking about depression, we can view antidepressants from several perspectives. We can say that they achieve an 80-percent cure rate, and that makes them sound good, because the number is high. Or we can say that they achieve an 80-percent cure rate as against a placebo cure rate of 20 to 40 percent. That's not so attractive from an advertising viewpoint, but it gives a truer picture of pharmacological effectiveness.

In recent years, as we have become more sophisticated, we have begun to look harder at this powerful "placebo factor." What does it involve? What is its mechanism? What kinds of people make the best "responders" to it? This becomes important not only for theory's sake, but because all of our studies are based on placebo. To what extent is real medicine important if the mind controls up to half of all therapy value?

We have already seen some of the delusions involved when we talked on pages 151–56 about the use of vitamins to cure schizophrenia. An improvement rate of 70 percent was shown while using chemical substances that were totally irrelevant! These rates were achieved by either suggestion or self-delusion. An enthusiasm may have been passed from healer to sick person. If the same experiment were conducted today, there would be no delusion, and hence no "miracle cure."

Here is a series of random observations, many of them gleaned from the pages of case studies, most of them well known to modern-day medical scholars, which better illustrate the power of the "placebo factor":

There is hardly an illness that placebo cannot affect. It can help 60 percent of all patients with headache, 25 percent with multiple sclerosis and about a sixth of all people who suffer from high blood pressure. The relief it offers will usually be temporary, but it *is* relief and it is often observable. In one recent review only people with epilepsy seemed to defy placebo's effectiveness.

Terminal cancer is not exempt from placebo. This case, quoted by Adolf Pfefferbaum vividly illustrates the phenomenon we are talking about:

> The patient described had generalized and far advanced lymphosarcoma [cancer of the lymph tissue]. He eventually became resistant to all therapies and developed anemia severe enough to preclude further radiation or chemotherapy. He had huge tumor masses, the size of oranges, in the neck, axilla, groin, chest and abdominal cavity. He was considered terminal by his physicians, but remained hopeful of a miracle.
>
> Then the reports of "Krebiozen" as a cure for cancer appeared in the newspapers. Although he did not meet the research criteria because of his poor prognosis, he was included in a protocol to test the efficiency of this compound.
>
> He was given the first injection on a Friday. His physician arrived to see him the following Monday expecting a "moribund or dead" patient. Instead, the patient was remarkably improved, and the tumor masses were half their original size. While none of the other patients in the study had improved, this patient recovered sufficiently to be discharged within 10 days.
>
> Within two months, newspaper accounts of Krebiozen failures began to appear, and the patient began to lose faith in this cure. He relapsed and was readmitted to the hospital in his original condition.
>
> At this point his physician deliberately lied, telling him that the drug was indeed effective and had merely deteriorated in storage. He was given injections of "fresh" drug, which was really only water.
>
> Recovery from his second near terminal state was even more dramatic than the first. Again he remained well for about two months, but then the final AMA announcement about Krebiozen appeared, declaring it to be worthless in the treatment of cancer. Within a few days the patient was readmitted to the hospital and died.*

*From *Psychopharmacology: From Theory to Practice*, edited by Barchas, Berger, Ciaranello and Elliott (Oxford University Press).

There are several studies extant showing that placebo injections are better than pills. Presumably the sight of a syringe and needle instills more faith in the patient about the treatment than an oral substance. A case in point is vitamin B_{12}. Remember when B_{12} shots were standard therapy? Of course they didn't do anything medical, but there were a lot of GPs who got great results with them!

There is a condition in medicine called angina pectoris—basically what most people would call a mild heart attack. Doctors used to treat this with an operation called an internal mammary artery ligation. It was simply the tying off of a chest artery—and it was absolutely useless in terms of real effectiveness. Yet it helped so many people that on a number of occasions doctors went ahead and did it anyway. They placed a suture, but they never tied it—and afterward the condition simply seemed to evaporate.

The attitude of the doctor seems to be highly relevant. There is a word in our profession—*iatrogenic*—which means any illness that has been caused by a doctor, such as drug addiction, anxiety, infection or allergy. A similar word that is related to placebo is *iatroplacebogenic*. It is used whenever a doctor or clinician acts in such a way as to create a placebo effect. We know that psychotherapy involves some placebo, and often the success or failure of its methods depends on the rapport the doctor has with the ill person. If he likes the patient, he tends to do well by her. If he finds her annoying, the success rate lowers. When there is good rapport, there is expectation—and the same principle applies when we are administering drug therapy.

I have mentioned before that in a number of instances a researcher has treated a patient with a perfectly good drug—and for a week or two his subjects have responded, showing all the signs of physical improvement. After a lapse of time the researcher has been told that the drug is not as promising as originally thought, and that the drug company has decided to withdraw the product, but that he should continue using it until all of his supply is gone. We have then noticed an astonishing change—the patients begin to suffer relapses. The only variable creating this effect is the soured attitude of the unwitting researcher.

Just as a doctor can radiate "healing," so too can the nurses and assistants who surround her. This has been shown in study after study, some of which have proven to be rather interesting. We know, for example, that when we're conducting a drug study there is great curiosity on the part of the staff members. They are eager to know which pill has the drug and which is the placebo being used for control purposes. An assistant may take the pills into a broom closet and taste them to see which contains the sugar product. And, as soon as the staff knows which is the placebo, the patients who have been taking it all claim to feel worse again.

The power of placebo can be so persuasive that it can completely reverse the power of chemistry. A perfectly good drug, if it's suspected to be worthless, will have none of the effects that are normally associated with it. Conversely, if you give a substance like ipecac—that is used to induce vomiting—to a patient who is suffering from nausea, and he believes it is medicine, he will often feel better.

We know from studies conducted during wartime that pain is largely psychic. A man wounded in battle can go without morphine, but the same wound at home would cause horrible agony. This has been interpreted by at least one investigator to mean that the presence of stress might increase placebo power. The soldier in battle is better fortified to deal with a pain that he has no control over. Put that same man in his friendly dentist's chair and give him the words, "This won't hurt a bit," and the minute he feels a probe on his teeth he will squirm until you give him Novacaine.

If some of this evidence seems contradictory—for example, does the presence of a "healer" create more pain or less of it?—it is simply because it *is* contradictory: we do not understand what creates the placebo factor. We have had many hypotheses, most of them wrong. We have tried to connect it to gullibility by saying that the person who is "trusting" is more likely to respond to ersatz medicine. This isn't true. Children are trusting, but when it comes to placebo, they are the same as the rest of us. Some get better and some don't—it has little to do with one's age or worldliness. Intelligence isn't a factor, either. Neither is race nor wealth nor status. The only thing that we feel reasonably sure of is that the healer's own enthusiasm is somehow implicated.

The reason I am taking the time to talk about this is that it drives to the heart of the mind-body construct. There *is* a connection between the two, and to ignore either one would be the height of foolishness. Throughout most of this book we have dwelt on the body. We have shown how the physical can affect the emotional. This is the drift of most modern psychiatry, and I have tried to show why there is plenty of reason for it. But simple answers are always inadequate. There's a mystery in our being that defies pure determinism. And this story of psychochemistry would be very lopsided if we didn't at least mention some countervailances.

It has long been recognized in both philosophy and medicine that the mind has power over our physical processes. This is a cornerstone of many religions, from Zen to Hinduism to the Christian Science movement. As early as 1775, Franz Anton Mesmer found that he could modify physical symptoms by "animal magnetism," or the power of suggestion. Mesmer's activities led to an enchantment with hypnotism, and hypnotism led us to Freud and analysis. So the history of employing the mind to change matter is as old and timeworn as the history of medicine.

In danger of being lost nowadays is the theory that the mind-body axis is a two-way avenue. We have become so enthralled with our chemical discoveries that we have all but forgotten the role that the mind can play. If it is true that our transmitters can affect our emotions, then it is just as obvious that the reverse is possible. It is like an endless loop, a chicken-or-egg cycle, and one can't assume that transmitters are the starting point.

Let's go back for a moment to the problems of anxiety. Anxiety, you'll recall, is a fear neurosis. Along with phobia and obsessive-compulsive behavior, it has proved highly resistant to the power of chemistry. There have been some fascinating studies of anxiety and phobia that show how emotions can affect our biology. They all tie in with the so-called learning theory, which has proven so essential to modern therapy.

It has been shown, for example, that a soldier in the midst of artillery fire in a wartime situation is likely to develop a wide range of symptoms, from nausea to amnesia to paralysis to speech defects. What is interesting about this is that, in the course of time, one of these symptoms is likely to dominate—usually that symptom which is most successful in relieving or avoiding the fear that he is feeling.

Let's say, for example, that when the first shell bursts, the soldier feels heart palpitations, dry mouth and nausea. All of these may be horribly uncomfortable, but they are no excuse for the avoidance of combat. Now let's suppose that, on top of these symptoms, he also experiences a strange paralysis. His trigger finger becomes immobilized. Try as he may, he can't get his gun to fire.

This is a symptom that psychiatry calls functional—that is, it has a purpose that is conveniently adaptive. The immobilized finger leads to the avoidance of fighting, and this is conducive to one's self-preservation.

Study after study in both animals and humans shows that when a subject is made to undergo punishment, the response (i.e., symptom) with the highest avoidance factor is inevitably the symptom that will come to predominate. Nausea begins to go away. Nor does the soldier complain about heart palpitations. The only symptom that will be left to bother him is the paralysis that forces him to stay in the foxhole.

From this it becomes apparent that when we talk about fear symptoms, we are actually talking about two phenomena: One is the fear, or anticipation; the other is the reward we get from avoiding it. Hysterical symptoms like paralysis or amnesia all seem to be based on this fear-and-reward phenomenon. And as long as you allow the symptom to flourish, there will be a notable reduction in the ravages of terror.

We can prove this hypothesis with experiments by taking two groups of rats and subjecting them to grid shocks. We will allow an avoidance mechanism for one group of rats, but the other group must simply endure what is happening. The actual shock is the same to both, but the physical results are entirely different. When the experiment is over and we perform a postmortem, we will find enormous lesions on the stomachs of the second group!

We can also gauge a change in transmitter activity. Animals that are allowed an escape route from punishment will show elevated levels of norepinephrine, while the others will show a lack of this transmitter family. Perhaps here is our link between anxiety and depression. Depression, you'll recall, shows low norepinephrine. And now we find that if you have no escape route, continuous pain can create the same neurological symptom.

This leads back to what we said about evolution—that sometimes these symptoms might actually be good for us. The theory is that we have built-in "on-off switches" that prevent us from struggling when struggling won't get us anywhere. The "wires" of this mechanism lead out to the environment. Our reactions are controlled by our minds, our experiences. Depression may simply be a state of anxiety in which we have become mentally convinced that we have no escape mechanism.

If you will accept for the moment that the definition of *mind* is "the accumulation of experiences that come from the environment," then you can see why there may be no great distinction between *iatroplacebogenics* and what we call will power. Both reside in the realm of the psychic. Both are invested with the power of healing. Whether we are talking about faith, witch doctors or nurses giving sugar pills, we are creating great chemical changes through such nonphysical avenues. We assume that these changes—or the messages that cause them—are being carried through the autonomic nervous system. This has meant, at least until recently, that we have also assumed that we are powerless to alter them.

But during the late 1960s a handful of researchers—each more or less independent from the other—conducted some experiments that would challenge this precept and restore to the psyche some of its lost charisma. One of these researchers, Barbara B. Brown, tells of her experiences in *New Mind, New Body*. They are worth recalling, if for no other reason than to reinforce our subplot of serendipity.

As Dr. Brown tells it, she was in the laboratory with a technician and a bright fifteen-year-old who was spending the summer as a helper. The youngster began by wondering whether his vivid visual images could be recorded so that they could be studied scientifically. The technician promptly rejected the validity of this, saying, "When I close my eyes, all I see is a field of gray."

They began to conjecture that if some people think in visual images and others don't, they should try to determine whether the *colors* of mental visual images might be reflected by differences in brain electrical activity. This seemed valid, for it had already been established that one's actual perception of colors is reflected in brain electrical activity.

Since they had had no experience with human brain waves, they implanted some electrodes in the brains of cats. Cats, it was presumed, had no sense of color, so it would be interesting to see if their brain waves reacted to color. They hooked the wires into recording instruments and then presented the cats with a series of colors. Lo and behold, there were distinct differences—the brain waves reacted to the various hues presented.

Next they decided to move on to humans. They found that different colors made different brain waves. They also found that people who were "color thinkers" had different traits from those who "thought grayness."

The next step in the experiment was pure coincidence. Since colors could affect a person's brain waves, they thought it might be fun to see if a person's brain waves could in turn be used to make a color selection. They chose as the color a soft shade of blue. They arranged it to be triggered by the *alpha* brain wave. This is a brain wave that is rather slow oscillating and is usually associated with deep relaxation.

The results of this experiment were truly remarkable. The subject started off with all kinds of brain activity. Naturally anxious at being wired like a stereo set, he was not very disposed to sending off alpha waves. Finally, however, some alphas came through, and as soon as they did, the blue light came on. He was then asked to describe for the researchers present what he was thinking and how he was reacting to it.

In subject after subject the results were the same. The blue light turned on with more and more frequency. The alpha brain waves began to dominate, and the subjects declared that they were totally at peace with themselves!

And this was how biofeedback got started. It got its name from computer technology, but the concept is as old as witchcraft and fakirism—only now we had the first tangible evidence of it.

There is nothing very new about the theory of feedback. It is really just an extension of traditional learning theory. For decades it was referred to as the *knowledge of results,* without which a subject could not learn to improve herself or himself. If we didn't see results, we would all be doomed to a random existence of trial and error. But, obviously, we have certain signs that we steer by, and some of those signs are physiologically imposed on us.

When we talked about the soldier with the immobilized trigger finger, in theory this reaction is not all that different from feedback. His "alpha wave" is his hysterical paralysis, and his reward (or "blue light") is the avoidance of combat duty. Thus the psyche, so often the captive, can turn the tables on physiology. It can call the shots, it can heal or destroy; and it can do this consciously as well as unwittingly.

I suppose one way to view medical history is as the continual displacement of the authority of healing. We began with that authority in the hands of outsiders, and we are moving toward the day when it may be vested internally. From priests and alchemists with the power of placebo, we displaced the authority into the hands of scientists. When Freud came along with his theories of analysis, the authority moved midway between the practitioner and the subject. Now, if biofeedback becomes the therapy of the future, the power to heal will become largely internalized. The patient will become her own practitioner, with IBM as both nurse and "Prayer Partner"!

Given the publicity it has received, I won't bother to detail biofeedback's achievements. I'll assume that you have read or seen on television some of the astonishing things that research is doing with it. Through feedback a person can alter body temperature, lower blood pressure or decrease heart rate by a kind of mental navigation, using brain waves and measurements as an internalized guidance system.

In psychiatry we have also begun using biofeedback, and it seems most attractive in combatting fear symptoms. A person with anxiety or a paralyzing phobia can be taught to control his physical reactions to it. Usually a therapist, working closely with the patient, will present the patient with a series of fear stimuli. Electrodes are attached to various body parts, measuring brain waves, skin temperature, heart rate and other changes. The patient, confronted by that which frightens him, tries to keep the needles from jiggling. It is a kind of game, like simulated flight tests, in which the object is to keep the craft on the landing beam.

We have had mixed results with these techniques so far, but the fact that we have had *any* success is an impetus for research. We need to know more about this method of treatment and how to achieve greater uniformity. Consider the advantages it has over drugs. Drugs can be used to eliminate fear symptoms. There's an old-time barbiturate called sodium amobarbitol, a structural cousin of phenobarbitol, which is very good at alleviating fear symptoms. The trouble is that fear is a necessity. A person who is fearless ends up in the hospital. It is all well and good to cure acrophobia, but not if it means you're going to become an Acapulco cliff diver!

Alcohol is also a very good fear fighter. Give a man a few drinks and he is afraid of nothing. He may become relaxed, outgoing, socially aggressive and may even tell the boss what he really thinks of him. The trouble is that when he gets in a car, he is equally unfrightened by threats on the highway. Cool, courageous, relieved of all anxiety, he becomes one of the most dangerous killers in modern society.

The potential advantage of biofeedback—and other techniques that are more or less allied to it—is that there is a conscious will, a sense of distinction involved, and we can govern our emotions according to circumstances. Also, of course, there is no fear of overdose, no side effects, no feelings of helplessness—we can be as pure and Calvinistic as we want without worrying about whether or not we are adulterating our biosystem.

All well and good. So why don't we use it? Why are we wasting our time on chemicals? Wouldn't it be a worthy goal for psychiatrists to teach all their patients how to utilize their alpha waves?

Unfortunately, the strength of biofeedback is also its weakness. It is because it *is* conscious that its usefulness is limited. Its effects are uneven, uncertain and temporary, and we have yet to verify its genuine efficacy.

Let's suppose for a moment that you can teach a person to lower blood pressure, which in fact is possible. By learning how to "flick" the appropriate switch, she can measurably control the walls of her arteries. In optimum conditions, with an ideal patient, you might teach her to do this without electrodes. Simply sit her down at a sphygmomanometer and—presto, chango—she becomes a healthy specimen.

Well, what have you accomplished? It might make for good vaudeville, but it is no indication that hypertension has been relieved. It may just mean that you have created a con artist—a person who knows how to get around blood-pressure tests.

The same is true for emotional disturbances. Given the possibility that you might consciously treat yourself, there is no guarantee—in fact, it seems rather improbable—that you could sustain this improvement on a day-to-day basis. Voluntary effort is therapeutically impractical. You would have to be a yoga master to make it work, and that is why biofeedback has remained limited to conditions for which short-term control is all that seems necessary.

There's another problem concerning all of this. Let's go back a few steps to take another look at the definition of *mind*. We defined it as being "the accumulation of experiences"—either present or remembered—"that come from the environment." That sounds pretty good—but how were they accumulated? What is this mystical, miraculous entity? Is it a puff of smoke? Is it a will-o'-the-wisp? Is it totally beyond all scientific inquiry?

You see, one of the problems is that some of the feedback advocates tend to romanticize "consciousness," as if only our minds were our true representatives, while the rest of the body is something that must be "conquered" somehow. You can see the problem—there is an implied duality. We will use "consciousness" to "control" the nervous system. It is "we" against "them," our body organs. We will "think" ourselves into robust healthiness!

But that may not coincide with the facts. The mind may not be distinct from the body. The body and the mind, whether conscious or unconscious, may both be part of the same reactor system.

At the risk of sounding materialistic, there is nothing in this world that might not be physical. Indeed, the whole thrust of scientific history has been to explain and diminish what was formerly thought to be "spiritual." The discovery of light waves ended years of philosophizing. Newton and Darwin punched holes in the miraculous with their theories. And so now, at least on a conjectural level, it is possible to derogate the primacy of consciousness.

If you think of our environment—what we experience with our consciousness—as sounds and objects translated into physics, then it is obvious that what we perceive as "psychic" is in reality a series of vibrations and light waves. These vibrations and waves, reaching the exterior of our bodies, energize our neurons through electricity and chemistry. The waves travel to the brain, through previously described mechanisms, where they are stored or imprinted by similar chemistry. The person in your memory is not really a person, any more than Johnny Carson actually comes into your living room. It is all done by ions and transmitters and colored by hormones at the command of the limbic system.

What this would mean is that the thing we call consciousness is no different in principle from the rest of our bodies. What philosophers (and psychiatrists) have been struggling with for centuries is simply an intricate network of transmitters and receiving units. The question of therapy becomes "point of entry"—at what stage in the process do you intrude with your "medicine"? Do you do it through the senses (as in psychotherapy) or at some later point, through surgery or chemistry? It is conceivable that the failure of psychoanalysis is not that it is erroneous but that it lacks precision. It may be too far removed from the point of malfunction, so that we are like electricians trying to fix things with a ten-foot screwdriver. Nevertheless, and

230

even with mittens on, we do succeed in relieving some mental problems, and we do this through an invisible physics whose means of healing is nonetheless chemical.

The same might be said of the powers of placebo. It might be a mistake to think of it as psychological. This implies that it is ethereal, ghostlike—a bundle of "forces" that only exist because of the names we give them. In fact, however, the attitude of the doctor—the message he or she communicates while dispensing the medicine—is also translatable into physics and biology, and we should not presume that there is anything mystical about it.

Finally, in reference to biofeedback, we may question the advantage of "self-control." This implies volition and self-supremacy, but in a mechanistic world these ideas may be meaningless. Worse than that, if we can control our own fates, and the method of that control is biological, it is not inconceivable that in some future world we could use similar principles to exert control over other people. In the beginning of this book I asked, "Who will play God?" It was a societal question, not really a personal one. But when you examine the skeins that psychiatry is unraveling, the question can summon up fears of apocalypse. In a world that is populated by machinelike organisms whose emotions themselves are biochemically determined, our belief that the mind is sacrosanct or holy makes as little sense as to say that depression is totally psychic.

Where does that leave us? That depends upon your bias. Is the glass half-full, or should we dwell on the dark side? Should we pray for the day when our minds are laid bare to us, or should we dread the destruction that could be implied in that? I really don't know. The people I treat as a practicing psychiatrist are in need of healing. Having embarked on this trail, I go where it leads me, but I do not welcome everything with unstinting enthusiasm. I view biofeedback as a potential ally and I am aware of the great new avenues it opens, but I do not believe in the cult that it has inspired, and I do not think it will provide all of psychiatry's solutions.

Taking the short-range view, one of the problems of feedback is that it has temporarily suffered from the blindness of enthusiasm.

231

We have become so excited that we can perform such miracles that it has led to a negligence of sound methodology. I believe we are in the process of rectifying this, but we badly need more controls, and better measurement. The intrusion of hardware into such a "soft" area requires some innovative substitutes for traditional placebo. We need, for example, effective miscues both for human brain waves and electronic responses. We need, in other words, the equivalent of sugar pills in order to measure this procedure's true efficacy. In addition, we need to know how to verify results better. Biofeedback is extremely subjective. The response we get one day fails to appear the next, causing a miracle of the moment to become irretrievable. I am certain that these problems will soon be vanquished. Considering that it took a century or better to arrive at good drug tests, we may view biofeedback as being just barely out of infancy, with the serious work on the subject only now beginning.

13

"The Mental Face-Lift"—
Improving upon Normalcy

One of the first things a psychopharmacologist will say is that the trend in recent years has been away from the "feel-good pill." We are now tailoring drugs to cure emotional and mental problems, and we are eliminating those that may be attractive to healthy people. The reason for this is patently obvious: Addiction and drug abuse have become major health problems, and we would like to believe that our profession is healing, not providing outlets for the world's bored and malcontent.

Nevertheless, beyond this platitude there are a number of exceptions, contradictions—and temptations. While we would like to think of our drugs as medicinal, there are areas in which the boundaries become questionable.

One of the continuing stains on the entire pharmaceutical industry—and, by extension, on we psychiatrists and doctors who work with it—is the unconscionable production of millions of products whose efficacy and value have been proven marginal. Barbiturates (let's name them), amphetamines and Quaaludes.

There is no justification for the abundance of these drugs. Their value is limited at best, at worst they can be killers, and the harm they have done far outstrips their usefulness.

The companies that continue to manufacture these drugs inevitably come up with but one rationale for them: There is someone, somewhere, who has been known to benefit from them, and to withdraw them from the market would be a denial of health care. We hear this argument applied to amphetamines, which are of extremely limited value in therapy. About the only excuse for prescribing them is in the treatment of hyperactivity or an illness like narcolepsy. Nevertheless, they continue to be produced by the thousands and millions. Eventually they find their way onto playgrounds and street corners. The companies that are mass producing these drugs cannot fail to realize the problem to which they are contributing.*

At the end of this book I'm going to be returning to this point, because it is one of those areas where policy has failed us. The drug industry has genuinely alarmed many people, who have become so frightened of drugs that they refuse to seek therapy. Suffice it to say that there are drugs whose abundance makes a mockery of the intentions of the majority of researchers, and their continued availability to the masses tends to undercut everything the rest of us are striving for.

This aside, it is generally true that the drugs of today have been better tailored than those of the past. They have been specifically produced to make sick people well and not to push normal people toward chemical pathology. THC, or *tetrahydrocannabinol*, is a good example. It is very effective at combatting glaucoma and reducing the nausea that accompanies cancer therapy. What makes it interesting is that THC is the active ingredient of the

---

*Interestingly, according to a recent article in the *Journal of the American Medical Association* (April 3, 1981), in the late 1970s Wisconsin decided to ban amphetamine prescription for all uses other than narcolepsy, hyperactivity or the psychiatric evaluation of depression. The result: average doses fell from 27,000 a month in 1976 to 800 a month in 1978—a 97 percent decrease. It was also found that of all the physicians practicing in Wisconsin, eight doctors were responsible for almost 90 percent of all amphetamine prescriptions! I am happy to say that two of those doctors have already been arrested and convicted in federal court.

marijuana plant. This puts it squarely in the disputed territory between viable medicine and a perceived sociological problem.

Marijuana, like all mood changers, creates many changes throughout the body. It lowers body temperature, changes EEG patterns, is an anticonvulsant and can depress certain reflexes. It can also effect the neurotransmitters. It reduces norepinephrine and elevates tryptophan. When you remember that tryptophan leads to drowsiness, this might explain one of the drug's chief appeals to its users.

Although marijuana was formerly a medicine, it fell into disfavor because of its attractiveness to healthy people. Ideally, medicine should not be too pleasant—or at least it should have nothing that leads to the abuse of it. We have experienced this problem with candy-flavored vitamins, which, although they taste good, should not be eaten like gumdrops. This has led to tougher restrictions in the packaging of health products for the nation's young people.

Because of the potential abuse of marijuana (it can create a number of long-term behavioral changes) it has been necessary to administer THC in a form that causes less euphoria. The form presently favored is a pill or capsule. The stomach takes the joy out of marijuana. This is because of gastric enzymes and juices that seem to metabolize the substance through different chemical channels.

The grapevine has it that Eli Lilly and Company will soon be marketing a THC "act-alike." Under the trade name Nabilone, it will be used to fight nausea but is said to produce little or no euphoria. It is ironic, perhaps, that a drug like marijuana must be introduced medically with so many safeguards, while older compounds that are more addictive and dangerous are liberally available, and few people challenge them.

When talking about the problems that drugs pose for healthy people, it might be wise to question our meaning. Indeed, it can be argued that many drug abusers are actually attempting a form of self-therapy. An analogy can be made with alcoholics, who are usually disturbed people. They won't see a doctor, they are afraid of medicine, so they turn to the bottle in an attempt to heal themselves. Anyone with any knowledge of chemistry knows that alcoholics have chosen the worst medicine possible, but that does not negate the strong possibility that alcohol might be used as an ersatz pharmaceutical.

And so it might be with many addicts and pill poppers. Too poor or ignorant or afraid to seek therapy, they turn to cocaine or barbiturates or "bennies" in a bungling attempt to be their own psychiatrists. It may be more than sheer coincidence that an age that is witnessing more depression among teenagers is also seeing more teenage drug abuse, as if the latter might inherently be the result of the former problem. If this is true, then when we talk about drug abuse it is possible that our concern has been misdirected. We should really be looking more closely at causes and less at the wrongness of the "medicines" being used against them.

Granted this viewpoint, it is nonetheless obvious that there are bad drugs, drugs that are mischievous, and that indeed we have yet to find any substance that can be used with impunity from unwanted side effects. This notwithstanding, the question arises: Does a healthy person also have a right to drug benefits? Despite our desire to limit drug use to the needy, might we not be tempted to try to improve "normalcy" with them?

In effect, here is the Huxleian bogeyman. There is the potential—and the pressure—to create a superrace. It triggers all the horrors of *Brave New World* and recalls ancient warnings about humans overreaching themselves. Certainly we see plenty of reason for alarm. When mankind tempts nature, it is a dicey gamble. We have seen the mess we have made of our ecology, and we quake at the prospect of being able to destroy ourselves.

But a question like this is definitely two-sided. Our notions of when nature should be inviolable may depend upon the circumstance. There are plenty of examples of nature being violated, and even the most romantic purist would not have had it otherwise.

At the beginning of my career, back at Worcester State Hospital, I worked with a doctor named Gregory Pincus. He was one of the pioneer researchers who gave us the birth-control pill, one of the most revolutionary drugs in the history of humankind. The Pill, of course, is a violation of nature. It does to the body what was never intended by preventing natural ovulation and creating a number of biochemical side effects. There are people in our society, in other respects antiscience, who would be outraged at the suggestion that they not use this chemical, declaring, and perhaps rightly, that it would violate their freedom and return women to the Dark Ages when they were thought of as chattel. It all depends upon one's point of view. What is sacrilege to one person becomes salvation to another. These discoveries are rarely unleashed upon society without society having already conferred its approval upon them.

We shall soon be facing this in psychopharmacology. We are approaching the age of "mental face-lifting," and, like surgeons before us, we will be dealing with the question of whether the methods we have developed should be restricted to sick people.

Let me give you an example of this. There has been a spate of recent research on the anatomy of the brain. It has been discovered that the left and right cerebral hemispheres have different functions in our behavioral and mental processes. The right side of the brain is the "visualization" side, which has to do with our *Gestalt* and space perception. It helps a person visualize in both real and abstract terms, which is the foundation of science, music and philosophy.

The left side of the brain is more verbally oriented. It is associated with instinct and putting things in context. It has been suggested that the left side is the barometer of our "social nature," helping us adapt to the community we live in.

Recently we have unearthed evidence leading us to believe that there are gender differences in the structure of these hemispheres: that men seem to have a more developed right side, while the female brain is leftward oriented. This could have sociological impact in that it will reinforce notions that the sexes are different, and that those differences extend far beyond reproductive functions. It will certainly not sit well with some feminist ideology.

Assuming that there are many people who will view these differences negatively—which I don't think any scientist would say is justified—such findings may be seen as a hindrance to progress,

237

particularly as interpreted by women who are goal oriented. It has taken hundreds of years for women to become accepted. Now, at long last, they are becoming doctors, executives. And here comes blind science, like a bull in a china shop, saying that women may suffer from some cerebral handicap!

If this proves true (and it is all terribly speculative), might it not be possible that we would want to correct this? Might it not be possible that there will be a groundswell of research to try to undo this anatomical injustice? And the impetus to do this will come from society. It might come from many of the same groups that idolize "naturalness." There is no one more revered than Mother Nature—except when it is perceived that she is pulling a fast one on us.

Inevitably in the course of our research on drug cures, there has arisen speculation about possible side benefits, which may not benefit the ill or psychotic but which may be attractive to people with no discernible handicap. We have already seen the lure in this direction with the impact of hallucinogenics. We have seen how a man like Aldous Huxley could first rail against science and then become rhapsodic about mescaline use. The attraction to expand has always been with us. We want to become greater, more intelligent, more talented. We are willing to attempt this even in the face of disaster, willing to risk prudence for a chance to be a superstar.

One of the side effects of the major tranquilizers is that they interfere with sexual activity. This is particularly annoying to many male patients, because there is a marked retardation in the ability to ejaculate. Upon first consideration this is seen as a nuisance. Science would like to eliminate this problem. After all, how can we lead disturbed people back into society if they are hindered or handicapped in their sexuality?

But as with all negative reactions, there is the opportunity for benefit, as in the case of Laborit's discovery of chlorpromazine. What to the rest of the world seemed an unwanted side effect he perceived as a wonderful discovery. Similarly, it has been suggested in medical literature that the dysfunction brought on by the

238

use of major tranquilizers, although usually considered undesirable, might prove beneficial in the area of sex therapy. If the drug could be modified, eliminating its mood effects, it might be useful on certain forms of impotence. Men who ejaculate prematurely might welcome the delay derived from the tranquilizers.

As a psychiatrist, my reaction is somewhat cautionary. Of all the sexual dysfunctions and hang-ups, the problem of psychological impotence is one of the easiest to cure by conventional therapy. And of all the forms of psychological impotence, the easiest to cure is the premature climax. So it would seem to me that to use a drug on this problem might be analogous to using a cannon as a flyswatter. Nevertheless, the temptation is obvious. And from the impotent male you could go to the sexually active. Through the use of chemicals you could sustain the libido, turning the act of coitus into an Olympic marathon!

I am not suggesting that anybody try this. You will not find Thorazine an aphrodisiac. But, at least in theory, it could be done, and all that is lacking is the social demand for it.

It has also been suggested that the hormone LH (the luteinizing hormone that we mentioned in our chapter on depression) is another potential remedy for impotence as well as a powerful contraceptive. In a British study middle-aged men who suffered chronic bouts of impotence were restored to normal sexual vigor after being injected with doses of LH. A Swedish study of twenty-seven women showed that if they inhaled the vapors of luteinizing hormone, it would curtail the release of other hormones essential for the completion of ovulation. This has led at least one wag to comment that LH may become the perfect marriage medicine. It perks up the man and protects the woman, and it might accomplish all this on one prescription!

There is another conceivable role for these chemicals. We could use them to destroy the sex drive completely, particularly in cases where morality might dictate that. There are certain societies in which the punishment for rape has been surgical castration of the offending party. In societies like ours this is considered barbaric, but we could achieve the same end through pharmacology. Dr.

Leo Hollister of Stanford University has raised this issue as a possibility. Prisons could be replaced by drugs, which are just as restrictive of the behavior of criminals.

Is this what we want? Again, it's a social choice. There has been a lot of criticism of our current penology system. Perhaps we would prefer a system of drug treatment that would obviate the need for Attica.

We have all seen instances in which powerful drugs have been used to expand the boundaries of normalcy. It is not uncommon for students in college to try "uppers" like benzedrine to help them through finals week. This is a foolish thing to do, but, leaving that aside, there is an issue at stake which I think is important. Like athletes with steroids, we are facing the day when drugs could be used to increase human brain power.

One of these drugs might be *ACTH*—short for *adrenocorticotropic hormone*. There is at least some evidence that, within limited parameters, ACTH can increase one's mental powers.

The body is made up of a series of loops. We have already talked about the limbic system. This is a loop that is contained in the brain and whose parts and subparts seem to control the emotional system. But there is a larger loop feeding off this circuit, which involves a number of glands and hormones. And it is within this loop—the adrenal system—that ACTH plays a vital function.

On top of our kidneys sit two cone-shaped glands, the adrenal glands. They store and synthesize three transmitters—dopamine, adrenaline and norepinephrine.

The adrenal glands are at the command of the limbic system, in particular a structure called the adenohypophysis. This is where ACTH comes from, and it is the "messenger chemical" that operates the adrenal glands.

You can see how vital this hormone must be to us. It is under the control of our "emotional coloring plant." But the gland that *it* controls is a primary source of the very substances that influence our emotional states!

Never was a lyricist more medically accurate than in those words to "The Windmills of My Mind." There are wheels within wheels, circles within circles, and the main goal of research is to try to locate the starting point.

ACTH has attracted attention not only because of its role in transmitter production but also because, by affecting the adrenal glands, it is a prime initiator of cortisol and steroid production. Steroids, as you may know, are one of the "miracle drugs." Synthetic steroids have a wide range of healing powers. They are also instrumental in muscle development and in various activities from sports to sexual functioning.

One of the surprises we have encountered is that ACTH—the messenger hormone that links all these wonders—seems also to be of vital importance in memory retention and our ability to concentrate. When you break down the components of ACTH to smaller fragments composed of amino acids, two of these fragments seem to be tailored expressly for brain activity.

You can give these substances to a rat, for instance, and they will make it, at least mentally, into a kind of "superrat." It will remember things better, learn things faster and be slower to forget whatever task is assigned it. When this was discovered, the natural response was to see what effect these substances would have on humans. This seemed particularly relevant to certain disorders such as retardation and senility.

The results are spotty, and there is some confusion as to the specific improvements, but the bottom line of these various studies is that there does seem to be an enhancement of mental powers. The subjects were able to concentrate better. They did not forget things—or at least not as rapidly. On a number of mental and memory exercises, their scores increased—and in most cases markedly.

That sounds good, but what about the rest of us? Can ACTH turn us all into wizards? Can it take a person with an average IQ and turn him or her into a Leibnitz or an Einstein?

Here the evidence is even less certain, but preliminary results have been more or less promising. In short-term studies of normal subjects, temporary improvements have been recorded. These improvements seem to center on visual retention, and they rapidly diminish in a fairly short period, but the fact that we see any improvement at all has ramifications for future societies. It is the first delicate toehold in the area of intelligence. It is the first sign we've had that IQ might be chemically changed. This in itself has social and political facets that are probably beyond our means to contemplate.

I should mention here that there are three major drawbacks that somewhat mitigate our general enthusiasm. One, as I've said, is that the effects are temporary, and we see no indication that we can permanently improve ourselves. A second major obstacle is means of administration. ACTH will not work in pill form. It must be injected intramuscularly if it is to get to the intended area.

The third major problem is that ACTH is very dangerous. It increases hormones that are extremely toxic. Like cortisone, it cannot be taken for long without causing susceptibility to infection and severe physiological deformities.

So as with everything else, we are long on promise and somewhat shy when it comes to delivering. ACTH may become one more blind alley—but as of this writing, it looks very promising.

Perhaps just as significant as the use of this hormone is the area of hypothesis it naturally leads us to. Because if ACTH can improve us mentally, what might this say about our human capabilities? Will we find, for example, that ACTH is more abundant in the minds of geniuses? Is this why some people can concentrate so well, while others are cursed with a short attention span?

It is reasonable to assume that in the years ahead we will be zeroing in on brain centers for human achievement—not just memory but also creativity, musicianship and what makes "gifted" or extraordinarily coordinated people. In theory these are all related to chemistry—a surplus or deficiency of various substances. Once we know what substances do what, we could conceivably give ourselves a talent or achievement "fix." There is a new invention that is making waves in the science world, a technique called *positron-emission tomography*. It is better known as PET, and it is related to the X-ray, only it is specifically designed to pinpoint brain activity. You can "label" a chemical with a traceable isotope, inject it into a patient's bloodstream, put the patient under a PET scanner and study the effects of the chemical's brain activity. Let's suppose, for example, that the chemical is glucose. Glucose is a source of energy. It tends to concentrate where its powers are needed, which means that it will be drawn toward the energized brain area. If you give a patient a shot of this substance and then tell him, for example, to raise his right arm, the PET scanner will show, as on radar, the exact location of the right arm's control center.

This method is being used in disease research, but is also potentially useful for schizophrenia. It could also be used to learn more about epilepsy or neuronal malfunctions like tardive dyskenesia.

And it could be used as well for studying the gifted. How interesting to be able to pinpoint the energy source when, say, Vladimir Horowitz looks at a Mozart concerto. Once you knew the energy source, you could devote all your research to the relevant millimeter. It is not improbable that in a relatively short time the mysteries of virtuosity would be unraveled.

This in turn leads us to speculate just how far *Homo sapiens* can go. I suspect there's a limit, but we haven't reached it, and right now it's like posing a "how high is up" question. I recall that when the four-minute mile was being broken routinely back in the mid-1960s, somebody asked the seemingly unbeatable Jim Ryun how low he thought the world's record might tumble. Ryun's answer was astounding to track fans. He thought he himself might better 3:50—and he supposed that with work, it was conceivable that a modern-day athlete might reach the 3:40 mark. Fifteen years later—a mere blink in history—a number of runners are crowding 3:40. What to yesterday's athlete seemed a miracle of achievement is today falling into the realm of the commonplace.

We are seeing our "limits" being exceeded all the time, and it is most notably apparent in the world of the athlete. The legendary marathon used to kill its participants, and now it is being run by octogenarians. Our knowledge of chemistry has, of course, been contributory. We know so much more about the human body— and of course drugs like steroids, amphetamines and sex hormones have played a controversial role in some of these "miracle" feats.

But not all these superstunts come out of a prescription bottle. There is a practice, for example, that team doctors call blood boosting, which involves replacing blood in a way that increases a young athlete's oxygen capacity. A recent article in the *New York Times Magazine* talked about a device called a *transcutaneous electrical nerve stimulator*. When applied to the skin, it creates electrical impulses that block the nerve signals from overstrained muscle areas. This sounds like it might be an equivalent to acupuncture, but they say that it is proving useful to athletes. And if you can block off body nerves, what might be the effects on the more psychic realms of endurance and competitiveness?

The point of this tangential discussion is that what can be done in athletics can be done in psychiatry. There is not enough difference between a brain and a calf muscle to preclude our ability to create superstar mental giants. Admittedly the brain is a great deal more complicated. It will take years to sort out all the myriad factors involved. But that is simply a problem of time; it is not a problem that requires any great knowledge breakthrough.

Whether this *should* be done is another matter. This is where society will have to arbitrate. Can we trust biochemists to control evolution, or would we prefer to keep it in the hands of natural selection? There is an ingrained taboo when it comes to human consciousness. We fear some rape, some ultimate invasion. I witness it daily, even with the patients I deal with—they have an inborn reluctance to let anyone get close to them. The mind is our final bastion. If we err, we are destroyed. We summon up images of robots and mad scientists. Do we dare permit this most Faustian of compacts, or would we prefer to live with our present blemishes?

I suppose the response of the average reader is "I'll live with mine—you can change all the others. Start with old Uncle Willie—he's mad as a hatter—then take care of the rapists, the muggers, the dope fiends and murderers." But that may not be the choice we are confronting. The knowledge that we're gaining holds marvelous attractions. And as I said at the beginning, can we

244

afford to be coy about it, given the propensity of societies to act so self-destructively?

Happily this will not be my question to answer. It may not be the question for any psychiatrist. We are but one small part of a mainstream of inquiry that includes all of existence and the laws that govern it. We began with the study of aberrant behavior. We wanted to know what made some people act "funny." After years of taxonomy, analysis and maze running, we have been brought face to face with electronics and chemistry. There have been others who have been following different avenues. There are surgeons and chemists and anthropologists, and last but not least, there is the world of physics, where energy and mass seem to dance in the hemisphere.

The further we advance, the more the sciences converge. Psychiatry and medicine seem to become one discipline. Chemistry and neurology and psychology and astronomy seem to ask the same questions as history and philosophy. When there is a "breakthrough" in one field, it suddenly becomes lionized. The word goes out through the universities: "Get into neurology, that's where the action is!" Or: "Forget about physics, it's all in biology now!"

In reality, of course, these advances are fleeting. Each discipline evolves through lurches and standstills. And the goal of each is to answer, "Why are we here?" and "Is there anything we can do to make our stay here more tolerable?"

At the beginning of this project, I believe I surprised my collaborator by saying, "You know, psychopharmacology is not the field of the future. If anything, it is only the field of the present. By its own definition it is self-eliminating." I am sure that he was discouraged to learn that this enterprise is not the equivalent of the discovery of the printing press, but that it is only part of a much larger endeavor and may someday become a mere footnote in history books. However, I sincerely believe this. Back in the 1950s when I first began to realize that analysis had limits, I shifted my research toward biochemistry, because psychopharmacology seemed to be so much more promising. Today, decades later, as I look toward the horizon, I believe that psychopharmacology will have lessening impact—not because there won't be important discoveries, but because new disciplines are likely to engulf the field.

You see, the ultimate goal of modern drug research is to lead us into a world in which drugs are not needed. This is the motive behind the study of brain chemistry and our attempts to unravel the mysteries of nature. Drugs as we know them are unacceptable. They are too imprecise, too grossly constructed. Only by knowing how *nature* makes drugs can we arrive at remedies that are physically appropriate.

I suppose we will always need remedies of some sort, even if they are derived from endogenous substances. Where there is life there is injury, there is the inevitable decay; and it is the nature of mortals to try to protect themselves. But drugs as we know them, drugs that habituate, drugs that create stupor and unwanted side effects will eventually, if researchers have their way, become as alien to society as treatment by crocodile dung.

And there is the outside chance, though it may seem remote, that nondrug therapy may yet gain ascendancy—that psychologists and behaviorists, through knowledge of brain mechanisms, may yet find a way to get us to heal ourselves. If it can be done through words, through rewards, through stimuli, if it can be accomplished through meditation or feedback, clearly that is preferable to ingesting any agent that exposes the body to trauma or injury. This, as I say, may seem light-years away—but then so was the attainment of the 3:40 mile. And there are many people working on it—in America, in Russia, on all five continents.

As the efforts of this research zero in on the "natural," and as endogenously produced substances become the researcher's paradigm, the focus shifts to the source of these substances, to the body itself and the origins of error. Psychopharmacology will not be the torchbearer for humankind's future; it is a transitional science, and is foredoomed to be the handservant of another discipline. For ultimately our condition—our diseases, our failures—is the manifestation of some deeper fallacy, an error or fragility so ingrained that it is the scientific equivalent of the

Original Sin concept. Researchers are already beginning to probe it, and psychiatry, in its own way, is closing in on it. We are doing so through drugs and neurological pathways that are leading us deeper toward the germ of our frailty. This subject has appeared in books and magazines, and you may have some dim awareness of its awesome importance. But I'd like to approach it from the angle of psychiatry and explain its significance to this thing we call consciousness.

I am talking about genetics.

14

DNA—The Origins of Error

Now and again throughout the course of this book, I have made reference to genetics—the "inheritance factor." I have talked about the likelihood of a predisposition to various conditions from depression to manic states. We have shown how schizophrenia seems to run in families. We have talked about depression as being more prevalent in females. We have implied that there is a serpent, some original "bad seed," that is imbedded in our makeup and is inherently transmittable.

The roots of this frailty are extended through history, running back to a period that precedes civilization. It precedes cavemen, dinosaurs—all life as we have come to think of it. "In the beginning," so it is written in the biologist's Genesis (there is likeness, after all, between *genesis* and *genetics*), "there was a bolt of lightning or some other phenomenon that created a cell where before there had been inanimacy." This may have happened about five billion years ago. This cell is called the *progenitor cell*. The ancestor of germs and seaweed and humans, it was basically similar to the cells in your body, with a few variations—a sort of "family resemblance."

From this progenitor came three lines of progeny. Two have remained in single-cell form, but the third divided and organized itself in such a way as to produce visible life forms. Somewhere along the line, something went wrong. Not *too* wrong, or none of us would be here. But some tiny particle, some submicroscopic substance, did not exactly act as we would have ideally wished it. Out of this aberration a number of frailties arose—baldness, myopia, dwarfism, heart disease. Many of these frailties were purely physical, but some resulted in behavioral and mental changes.

When people decided to study these behavioral oddities, this is where psychiatry came in. We cataloged them, analyzed them, tried various remedies on them—and finally stumbled on the use of chlorpromazine.

Research from that point on has been the subject of this book. The use of psychoactive drugs led to the discovery of transmitters. Transmitters led to the uncovering of mechanisms that seemed to be associated with psychopathology. But beyond these mechanisms there are also fundamental errors. Something went askew in the earliest development. It is the goal of psychiatry, our ultimate destiny, to uncover and correct these most elemental fallacies.

To do this we have to know what we are looking for. We had to know, first, the behavioral consequences. We had to see depression as distinct from mania, and mania as distinct from schizophrenia. Once knowing this, we had to examine neurochemistry. We had to see which malfunction could be paired with which illness. Only after that could we begin our search for the genes responsible for each chemical misfiring.

Obviously we are just starting our research into this last stage, and there are many questions we have yet to find answers for. Is it an overabundance of "X" that we're talking about, or is it a deficiency of "Y," which is X's antagonist? This is a matter of plodding and research, and also a matter of increased technology. With better tests, better machinery, we should be able to uncover the answers we're looking for.

It has been said that science is the discipline of measurement. Measurement implies the perception of quantity. There is no such thing as a qualitative difference when we're talking about someone who is neurotic or has mental problems.

This does not mean that the concept of quality is valueless. Obviously there is a difference in a painting by Van Gogh and the scribblings of a child with a box of Crayolas. But it is the duty of science to take this difference and reduce it to terms that are objective and measurable. This is not easy, and it is sometimes unpopular.

If I could summarize all that we have learned in this book, it could perhaps be reduced to a simple diagram. The diagram would not be complete; it would not be quite adequate; but the schematic structure might look something like *Figure 1*, page 251.

From this you can see that there are four potential trouble spots. Each of these can have a variety of problems. This is admittedly an oversimplified view, but it is important that we can at least put some finite boundaries on it.

1. There may be problems in transmitter manufacturing. In the case of depression, there may be too little. In the case of schizophrenia, there may be too much—particularly of dopamine, which is made in the midbrain area.

2. There could be problems with the MAO, whose role it is to destroy the transmitters. In the case of depression there may be too much, in the case of schizophrenia there may be too little of it.

3. There could be a problem in the receptor-site area. This is our theory of nerve cell "sensitivity." Too many receptors, or perhaps too few of them, could influence the neuron's "excitability."

4. Finally there's the possibility of a malfunctioning inhibitory system. This is the system that keeps cells from firing. It uses substances like GABA and glycine to tell the originating cell to stop firing.

Having identified the trouble spots, we now come to causes, where the going gets trickier, because there are a number of

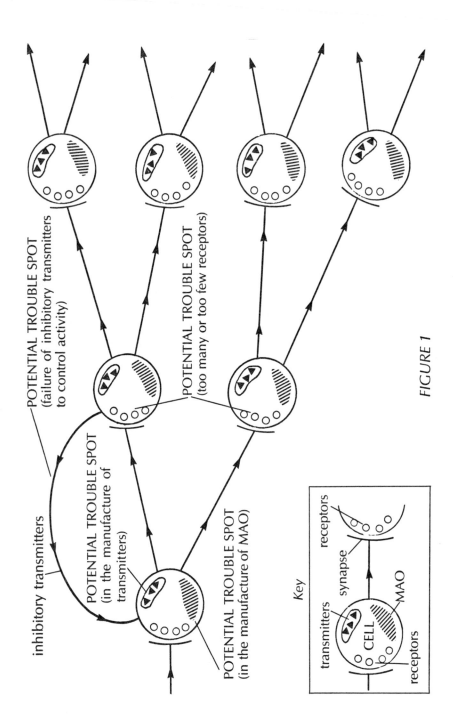

POTENTIAL TROUBLE SPOT
(failure of inhibitory transmitters
to control activity)

POTENTIAL TROUBLE SPOT
(too many or too few receptors)

inhibitory transmitters

POTENTIAL TROUBLE SPOT
(in the manufacture of
transmitters)

POTENTIAL TROUBLE SPOT
(in the manufacture of MAO)

Key

transmitters
receptors
synapse
CELL
MAO
receptors

FIGURE 1

reasons these areas may malfunction, and they go right to the heart of all cellular activity.

The human cell is an extraordinary environment. It could almost be compared to a colony of honey bees. There is a "queen," there are "drones," there is communication, and all the various workers seem tirelessly dedicated.

If you could take a journey inside a cell, you would find it similar to a duchy or feudal system. It contains a "castle"—or *nucleus*—in which lives the "queen" surrounded by an environment that we call the *cytoplasm*. Within this environment there are a number of peasant types, simple little entities we call the *ribosomes*. It is they who gather amino acids and synthesize them into proteins. Perhaps they are to become part of a blood vessel, or a piece of skin, or a particle of enzyme. It all depends on the cell's location and what the "queen" has decided must be built that day.

Before this analogy gets too anthropomorphic, I should warn you that these characters are not very humanoid. In fact, they are like nothing you have ever seen, unless you spend your days in a laboratory. Even then you may not have seen them, since some live beyond the reach of the most powerful microscope. But we know that they are there, and through various assays we can pretty well determine the size and shape of them.

I have often been struck by the unusual likenesses that exist between natural and manufactured objects. It is as if, given the infinite variety of existence, there are only so many shapes that are truly functional. You have probably seen drawings in which molecular structures resemble Tinkertoys. Well, those illustrations are accurate—that is what they look like. The inventors of Tinkertoys were just copying the physics books.

In trying to describe the shape of the "queen," it may help if we think of her as somewhat reminiscent of a toy called a Slinky. A Slinky is a spring that children play with, which "walks" downstairs and performs other amusements.

The "ruler" of a cell looks somewhat like that. It is a twisted little spring made of sugar, phosphates and nucleic acids. Acually it is *two* springs, their spirals entwined, as if you had meshed two Slinkies to form a double density.

We call this construction a *double helix*. *Helix* is simply a word meaning "spiral." We call the "queen" *deoxyribonucleic acid*—or, more affectionately, the DNA molecule.

The history behind the discovery of this entity is as long and tortuous as any in science. It goes back to an Augustinian monk named Gregor Mendel who performed the first experiments in the mid-nineteenth century proving the existence of genetics. The life forms he worked with were very primitive. He cross-bred certain plants and vegetables. He noticed that the offspring came out different, and that the qualities of both parents were discernible in their progeny. This led to the discovery of the existence of *chromosomes*. The chromosome, to Mendel, was the "formative element." It dictated the difference between, say, white and red flowers, which, when bred together, would produce a motley color.

All well and good, but when you are dealing with plant life, you are only dealing with one or two chromosomes. The potential for difference is not that dramatic, and it certainly wouldn't account for all the variety in animal life. It took many years before science got wise to this. Chromosomes were obviously an inadequate answer. There must be something *within* the chromosomes that dictates each of life's infinite differences.

The discovery of this "something" did not come quickly. It took a number of biologists and a number of experiments before, in the early part of the twentieth century, the existence of *genes* was finally arrived at. Now it became known that this thing called the chromosome was actually shaped like a string of sausages. And each of its links was a separate gene, which, when combined with another, produced a trait or quality.

There are about 100,000 gene types in each human body. Each is responsible for thousands of cell structures. The number of cells reaches up into the many billions, with a large proportion crammed up in our craniums. The genes are contained within 48 chromosomes, half from the sperm and half from the ovum. The genes pair off into 50,000 traits, which we exhibit in infinite combinations.

It is not unreasonable to argue, as science does, that everything we are is imbedded in this gene structure. Our strengths, our weaknesses, our talents, our deficiencies are all derived from the links in these sausage strings. Evolution suggests that environmental factors have served to help certain traits predominate. But our hold is tenuous, since we all have frailties, and the environment is something we must struggle to cope with.

Once we nailed down the existence of genes (which replicate, by the way, from the time of conception; so that when we are talking about genes and talking about body cells we are talking about things with a similar infrastructure), another problem quickly presented itself: How do the genes know what they are doing? How do they remember what their roles in life are?

In 1953 an American named James D. Watson, with a British collaborator named Francis Crick, published a one-page article in the journal *Nature* that was to strike the world like a bolt of lightning. "We wish to suggest a structure for the salt of deoxyribose nucleic acid," the article began, rather unpromisingly. "This structure has novel features that are of considerable biological interest." The article went on to describe a structure, like two entwined spiral staircases, held together by regularly spaced "steps," so that each side of the spiral is connected with the other side. It looks like *Figure 2*, page 255.

This, of course, was the "double helix." And this is what our "queen" is shaped like. Each segment of spiral is separately encoded by the nitrogenous "steps" that hold the two sides together.

The reason I called forth the image of Slinkies is that DNA has certain springlike qualities. Like a spring, it can coil into larger spirals, twisting itself into all kinds of knot shapes. We call these configurations *supercoils*. Basically, they are the result of sophisticated "packaging." The more coils that can be packed within the DNA structure, the more messages that can be contained within a very small area.

FIGURE 2

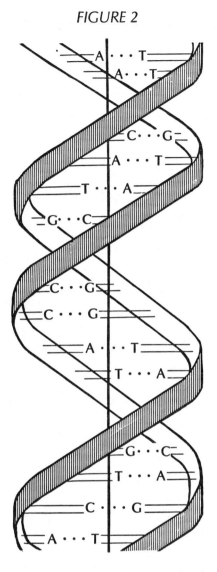

A highly schematic view of how DNA looks, in theory. (In reality it is much more complicated.) The spirals are made of sugars and phosphates. They are connected by horizontal steps split in half. The steps are made of adenine (A), cytosine (C), guanine (G) and thymine (T). A is always paired with T and C with G. These combinations form the genetic codes.

Like the queen of a castle, the DNA molecule is more or less prisoner of its own unique status. It cannot get through the walls of the nucleus to communicate directly with "serfs" in the cytoplasm. To do this the "queen" needs a "lord"—a royal ambassador who can act as press secretary. This royal ambassador can leave the nucleus and tell the ribosomes exactly what's wanted of them.

This agent is *ribonucleic acid*. It goes by the acronym of RNA. It is exactly the same as DNA but with some segments omitted so that it can leave the nucleus.

Let's say DNA has a message to give. It wants to build some additional protein. The organ it inhabits seems a little restricted, and it wants to tack on some additional tissue. The first thing it does is reproduce itself. It makes a molecule of the very same structure and then, through the use of enzymes, some segments are deleted so that the molecule can pass through the walls of the nucleus.

The RNA exits, carrying DNA's message, and goes out into the cytoplasm, where it encounters a ribosome. The RNA touches the ribosome with one of its encoded spirals—in this case a spiral that commands the acquisition of tyrosine. The ribosome reacts by sending out for tyrosine. The RNA then rearranges its position. It touches the ribosome with another message, to get glycine or phenylalanine, or whatever else is called for.

So you have all these incredible activities going on within a space that can only be measured in light waves, and they are going on in every part of the body, including the aforementioned "potential trouble spots." What if there's a flaw in one of the DNA segments? What if the RNA bungles its assignment? What if the carriers bring in too much glycine, and the ribosome has more than it is equipped to deal with? The variables are multiple. There are inhibitory molecules whose role it is to guard against surplus. What if one of these begins to malfunction? What if some toxin invades the whole cell mass?

The art of measurement . . . You see, the view that we're taking is that there are so many measurements, so many ingredients, that they don't have to be off by more than a smidgen to wreak wholesale havoc on our mood or our mental functions. And they don't have to show up immediately, either. They can lie dormant. They can build up slowly. Atom by atom, chip by chip, they can create a fissure that will someday give way on us. *The art of measurement* . . . It's analogous to bridge building. There are trusses, I-beams, asphalt, concrete, and each of these has numerous ingredients that can dictate its strength and flexibility. You build a bridge properly, and thousands of cars and trucks pass over it. It all looks perfect to the naked eye; no one can see the separation of molecules. *The art of measurement* . . . Tyrosine . . glycine . There could be too much, like the sand in the concrete. And slowly, invisibly, the foundation could granulate, waiting for the first heavy wind or the next rainstorm.

And that's how it is when we confront the environment. Something upsets us. We are mentally blind-sided. And like the bridge that begins to creak and shudder, there's a silent snap, some break in the cell structure.

Fortunately for us, nature usually has remedies. For one thing, we have many duplicates. Two lungs, two kidneys, two eyes, two brain hemispheres—we cannot complain that we have been cheated in the parts department. Nature is also good at finding alternate solutions. If something fails, nature works around it. Even behaviorally we learn to adapt ourselves—through repression, amnesia, conversion and other patterns.

Perhaps we have built-in genetic safety nets. Perhaps it takes more than one gene to create a pathology in us. Perhaps it takes a number of genes, all malfunctioning in combination. In psychiatry we call this the *polygenetic* theory. In its various details it is statistically complicated, but basically it says that out of "X" conceivable errors there must be a number that have happened before we can get, say, schizophrenia. Suppose there are six genes that can create this illness. Perhaps all of us have one or two in our makeup. But perhaps it takes three or four or five before we develop a discernible proclivity for the illness. Now let's suppose also that there are four nerve areas where these carrier genes would have to be functioning. It could be that we could tolerate a "misfiring" in one and show very few changes in our outside behavior. It may take two before we would show any signs—and the character of our behavior would depend on the nerve sites. It would also depend on which of the genes was responsible for the problem in that particular area.

It might also be that we are carrying other genes that have created a weakness in another nerve area, but as long as we are facing no untoward pressure, the system holds up and we act reasonably normally.

But now, like the bridge, we may face the first windstorm. Or it could be but the last of a series of windstorms. Some structures give at the very first pressure, and with others it takes repeated punishment. Now the strands begin to give way. One causes autism, another delusions. A third one snaps, causing paranoia, and a fourth triggers frenetic giggling. Pretty soon the subject will find himself hospitalized. He will be chastised and branded as schizophrenic. He will have all the same qualities of the "mad-man" or "lunatic" or those poor souls who used to be burned as "witches."

Yet there is nothing about him that is all that different! He is not inhuman. He is not inferior. His only "crime" was an error in quantity—too much or too little in too many junction boxes. One change in one factor and he might have been normal. He might have been bald or stunted or cross-eyed. He might have been fat or walked with a limp, but he would not be branded as a leper or a monstrosity.

And what has caused this? Was there a virus? Was there something that altered the very first parent cell? When that cell divided, did it divide its infirmity, spreading error and tragedy throughout the whole biosystem?

One of the happier things about medicine is that you don't always need to know ultimate causes. It helps, of course, and we'd like to know them, but we often find cures in the midst of our ignorance. We don't know the causes for manic-depression, but we are grateful anyway, because we know how to treat it now. We have lithium, and it is quite dependable, and we feel relatively safe against this frightening mental ailment. We have phenothiazine, and that helps schizophrenia. Maybe we'll get lucky and discover some virus at work. Once we do we can develop a serum and get rid of the illness through inoculation.

A few years ago a patient I was treating, a depressed young man who was also remarkably intelligent, asked me, "What's it all about? What are we doing here?" He had a religious bent—I believe he was Catholic—and he seemed often to ponder such cosmic conundrums. I believe he was asking, "In view of my inadequacies, what is the meaning of life on this planet?"

To be perfectly honest, I don't know. I am as ignorant on that score as any other mortal. And it is certainly not for any doctor or psychiatrist to intrude in the area of theology. But I had read a science-fiction book once in which the author suggested that DNA was our master. DNA, said the author, had its own secret motives, and we are but one of the agents it works through.

"Perhaps we're here to serve DNA," I said to my patient. "After all, it is the one thing that will always survive. No matter what life form it chooses to inhabit, it goes on and on, endlessly replicating."

Well, I was somewhat astonished to find out later that this young man had gone and told all his friends: "Dr. Rosenblatt says that he's found God! It's deoxyribonucleic acid!"

Let me try to repair this: Whatever DNA is, I do not think it's God. It is but one more link in a great chain of being, the beginning of which is still lost in obscurity. But professionally speaking, *biologically,* it is a significant new star to guide our ship by. It is still very distant, very clouded in guesswork, but it gives us new daydreams to feed our enthusiasm.

During the last few years there has been a surfeit of literature on the science of gene splicing—making new life forms. We call this phenomenon *recombinant DNA,* meaning DNA that has been altered to produce different cell life. We can do this now. You have probably read about it. We can take DNA out of a tiny bacterium, cut it open with the use of enzymes and insert a slice from some other genetic matter. The result is the creation of an entirely new gene. The gene will have whatever traits we dictate, and it will go on replicating—reproducing—creating an organism of a whole new character.

This can be a frightening fantasy. It summons up images of *The Andromeda Strain*—malignant bacteria, horrible mutations, things that threaten to destroy humanity. And the speed of this process is awesome to contemplate. Within an hour or two it can create whole colonies—billions and billions of strange little progeny. We have heard that these might be useful for industry. We could create a bacterium that could clean up an oil spill. We could use DNA to make antibiotics—or floor wax, or shoe polish, or to mine silver or copper ore. The visionaries among us see DNA as a labor force. The skeptics see it as a frightening new enemy. I would not be surprised if both the United States and Russia were studying its implications for warfare.

But from a healing standpoint—which is what I am concerned with—DNA might yet prove an ally. In some far-off land, a kind of medical Oz, it may spell the end of dreaded psychosis.

Let's suppose, for example, that a few years from now we have sorted out the knots in our neurotransmitter theories (reality, of course, is rarely so generous; we are as likely to have discovered new complications); let's suppose that we have nailed down all the trouble spots and have a clear idea of the chemicals involved in them, and that genetic science has progressed sufficiently that we know exactly which genes are responsible. Now let's suppose further that certain allied disciplines—such as statistical science and epidemiology—have evolved to the point that we can examine a patient and determine the likelihood that he is a candidate for schizophrenia. Let's suppose that our dreams have come true. Let's suppose all these unsupposables. You can see where the miracle of recombinant DNA would make all other answers seem pale in comparison.

We could take a young woman who has a predisposition toward schizophrenia and explain our concerns about her having a baby. Perhaps we would then suggest a simple gene splicing to make sure the child keeps the proper dopamine level.

This could be done on an outpatient basis. We would simply

extract an ovum from her uterus. In a lab we would culture a virus-type agent with a gene inside that would correct the deficiency. If the problem was, say, receptor formation, we would culture a gene that made proper receptors. Or if it was determined that the problem had to do with glycine or GABA, we would utilize a gene that corrected this fault.

We would then introduce this virus to the ovum. This is literally all we would have to do with it. The virus would carry the corrective gene and implant it in the ovum's cell structure.

Now half the cells of the offspring-to-be have a corrective genetic material inside of them. Twenty-four of the forty-eight chromosomes carry built-in insurance against schizophrenia.

Once the sperm implanted the ovum, the corrective material would begin to replicate. It would replicate in every cell in the egg, encoding its message on every DNA molecule. Of course, the cells we are concerned with are only the brain cells, but there are inhibitor genes that make sure that your cells only produce material that's appropriate for each body area.

Thus we can foresee a day when the scourge of psychosis is completely eliminated from this planet—a day without Freud; a day without drugs; a day without shock treatments or mental wards. When this might come—or even *if*—is anybody's guess; it's beyond all prediction. We have seen too many theories, too many disciplines that seem to rise in optimism, then sink to confusion again. Physics once seemed to be the answer to everything. It is now confronted with baffling enigmas. Even mathematics, that most "pure" of all sciences, seems to have fallen far short of the goals it once set for itself. I am too humble to believe that we psychologists are any exception. This is suddenly being touted as The Age of Biology. And it *is* a great age, and I have been proud to partake in it, but I am not deluded that we are about to find paradise.

Rather, what we are doing is simply crossing a threshold. We are leaving one era and entering another. People have been doing this since the world began, and it is only history that can pass sound judgment on it. What concerns me more are certain short-range obstacles. I can't predict into the twenty-first century. That century will have its problems, and they will probably be big ones, and whatever we have already done may be perceived as naive then. But I can say for certain that even the daydreams that *we* have, even our modest hopes of improved pharmacology are being threatened by a complex of problems that could become the equivalent of the oil or energy crisis. I am talking about drug regulations, and I am also talking about the Food and Drug Administration. Like all doctors nowadays, I have my own views on this—but it will take a new chapter to present them coherently.

15

The FDA—Some Political Nettles

In 1937 an American drug company—the Massengill Company in Bristol, Tennessee—made a miscalculation of such horrible proportions that the medical industry still bears the scars. It was the year after the discovery of a miracle called sulfa drugs. Sulfa was the first great antibacterial agent. It had been discovered abroad in 1936 and brought to this country, and drug houses everywhere were scurrying to market it.

Thirty-one years earlier, in 1906, Congress had passed the first Pure Food and Drug Act. It was a landmark act, a great piece of reformism stirred by scandalous conditions in both the drug and the meat industries. Yet it was very broad and rather loosely constructed. It simply guarded against gross impurities. It was certainly not equipped to handle the technical explosion that was soon to descend upon the burgeoning drug industry.

To the folks at Massengill the arrival of sulfa drugs presented a wonderful opportunity. They could jump into the market while it was still young and growing and make a great deal of money from an eager client list. There was no necessity to test this substance.

The Europeans had proven that it was efficacious. Besides, there was nothing in the Pure Food and Drug Act that said a medicine had to be tested before distribution.

So the decision was made to market sulfanilamide. But Massengill's next decision was to prove calamitous—and it was to change forever the practice of medicine making.

"What if we made it a *liquid?*" they asked themselves. "That would give us an edge on competitors. There are a lot of people who don't like pills, but if you made it like syrup it would probably prove popular."

They instructed a chemist to set about doing this. He willingly obliged—it was an innocent assignment. He took sulfanilamide and mixed it with alcohol, and they all stood back to see what the result was. The sulfa refused to dissolve in the fluid. The chemist decided that the problem was the alcohol. He looked around for an alcohol substitute and settled on a substance called diethylene glycol. Diethylene glycol is what we call a demulcent. It is a colorless liquid in the glycerine family. Glycerines are used in many medicines, including ointments, lipsticks, skin balms, and other remedies.

He tried this agent, and the results were wonderful. Now the sulfa was totally soluble. They added some coloring, some tasty fruit flavoring, and got a very palatable medicine.

Hundreds of bottles of this miraculous new cure-all began pouring out of the Massengill chemical plant. For the most part they went to places like Atlanta and Tulsa, cities in the southeastern corridor.

The first reports came out of Tulsa: SIX PEOPLE DIE AFTER SWALLOWING MEDICINE! But soon they were coming out of other towns, too—horrible stories of writhing fatality.

In Chicago the American Medical Association, hearing of these deaths and of their link to the sulfa product, immediately requested that the Massengill Company send them some samples from the company's inventory. Massengill complied. They had nothing to hide. They were totally within the bounds of both ethics and protocol, and whatever else you could lay at their feet, you could not accuse them of criminal activity.

What the AMA found was to shock America. The bottles did not contain medicine at all. You see, sulfanilamide mixed with diethylene glycol becomes the chemical structure for automobile antifreeze!

One hundred and six people died from this error. There were calls for a congressional investigation. The president of Massengill defended his company—but the chemist, distraught, committed suicide. In the months that followed it became clear to everyone that the Pure Food and Drug Act was no longer adequate. In 1938 the law was revised, and the result was the Federal Food, Drug and Cosmetic Act.

The Food and Drug Administration, or FDA, became the watchdog of a variety of elevated standards: more honest advertising, display of warning labels, withdrawal of unsafe drugs from the marketplace. Most important, the law made it mandatory for drug companies to test their products for safety; and the FDA was given powers of enforcement that far exceeded that of most other regulatory agencies.

Ironically, the one thing that was still *not* required was that a company test each drug for "efficacy." In other words the drug would have to be safe, but it was not required that it do any good.

In 1957 a drug company in Germany, Chemie Grünenthal, came out with a cold remedy with the trade name Grippex, an over-the-counter medicine like Coriciden or Dristan. It was soon found to be highly sedative. Somebody decided to reformulate the marketing. They changed the name from Grippex to Contergan and reintroduced it as a kind of tranquilizer.

Contergan became a popular medicine. In Germany you didn't need a prescription for it. In countries like Switzerland, Italy and England, it was more controlled, but it was still widely distributed.

In 1961 an application to sell this substance was received by the FDA in Washington. It landed on the desk of Frances Kelsey, a young clinician who had recently been hired there. At this point the story becomes somewhat ambiguous. Dr. Kelsey claims that the results of some animal tests genuinely aroused her medical skepticism. Be that as it may, approval was delayed. The papers sat in the FDA pending file, creating a unique example of bureaucratic lethargy actually averting a calamity that could have been mind-boggling.

Contergan, or "K-12" (its experimental label), had already been approved in forty-six countries. And while the forms sat gathering dust in Washington, reports from Europe began to crop up in literature—reports of first one birth deformity, then ten, then a hundred. Soon it had swelled to an epidemic. In the end, K-12—which we call thalidomide—claimed thousands and thousands of newborn infants.

In the aftermath of this horrifying tragedy, new teeth were added to the US drug code, making it necessary for drug manufacturers to prove that a drug had medical efficacy. In addition, the FDA established an arduous review process to examine all drugs introduced since 1938. This led to a number of restrictive measures against "high abuse" items like barbiturates and sedatives.

As for Dr. Kelsey, she became a heroine. The US government gave her a medal—surely the first time in American history that a bureaucrat was honored for procrastination!

What, you may ask, is the point of all this? Well, it is simply that we are now faced with a predicament. And to understand the nature of our problem, it is necessary to know the steps that led up to it.

As a doctor, I suppose I am naturally conservative. Actually, politically, I am probably liberal. I have a strong desire to see society improved, and I have been known on occasion to hope that government will do this for us. But as a practicing psychiatrist, I am increasingly dismayed at our federal bureaucracy. I am reasonably convinced that the FDA has become the unwitting victim of its own success story.

Let me hasten to say that in this hierarchy none of the components is completely blameless—neither the scientists upon whom our knowledge depends nor the drug companies that finance so much of the research. In this book I have painted a picture of heroics. We have seen "dedicated scientists" making

266

"great discoveries." But there is another side of this profession we are in, and it is one that isn't seen on television medical shows.

Not long ago you may have read about a prominent professor who was slighted by a grant committee and who allegedly retaliated by turning his laboratory into a factory for producing cocaine and heroin. Before that there was the story about the dean of a medical school who had been forced to resign under shadow of scandal, and, earlier still, a Sloan-Kettering researcher who had been discovered falsifying the results of some rat tests. These things do happen. I won't deny it. I have seen cases of falsified and plagiarized research, I have seen scientists like our midwestern doctor with his endorphins who have confounded their colleagues with imprudent enthusiasm. And there are many other scientists who are probably glory seekers. They will perform tests on anything, regardless of logic. If they fail, no harm done; if they succeed they are heroes, and everyone will say they are incredible geniuses.

The politics of science is very seductive. It can lead you to follow the false hypothesis. It can lead you to cling to some patent absurdity because you have invested so much of your time and enthusiasm in it. It can take a well-meaning man and make him an "unscientist" who will continue to give niacin to cure schizophrenia, claim to see illness in the chemicals in hair or try to cure phobia through outmoded analysis.

Then there are the big pharmaceutical houses. There the motive is money, not glory. They are extraordinarily jealous on behalf of their coffers, and they will do many of the same things we see in other businesses. There have been cases in which, while testing some product, a company has come up with negative findings. Legally they are committed to report those findings, but the reports have been known to get "lost" in a file somewhere. In the course of our research, while talking to representatives of various companies, we saw their subjectivity firsthand. In a couple of cases we faced vague threats when it seemed that we might say something too damaging.

So, again, we can appreciate the forces at work here. Science is not an ivory tower. And you can see why the people at the FDA must pick their way warily among the "gospels" presented to them.

But let's look again at the history of our drug laws. I believe that the dates tell the story eloquently. And when you look at the facts of the past two decades, that story unwinds into a monotonous litany.

In 1936 sulfa was discovered in Europe, and within a year Americans were using it. One hundred and six people lost their lives, but not because there was anything wrong with sulfanilamide.

Two decades later we had stronger laws. This time, with thalidomide, the time lag was a full five years. What the world had been using since 1957 came to the attention of Americans during the term of John F. Kennedy.

Thalidomide was bad, and the FDA was correct. If it had gotten loose in a country like ours, the number of victims would have been incalculable. But now let's look at our more recent drug history. Take, for example, the antidepressants. We are still using drugs that are twenty years old, with very few new compounds available for marketing. There's one new compound that I mentioned, by the name of *maprotiline*. It is just in the process of being launched, and a look at its history is very illuminating.

Maprotiline (brand name, Ludiomil) is an antidepressant. It is a member of the family of drugs called tetracyclics. It was discovered in Europe in 1962 and was available there not too long afterward. A search through the available American literature shows no mention of maprotiline until the early seventies. In other words it took almost ten years before American doctors were even aware of it.

During the next eight years there was a scattering of research on maprotiline. We still lack widespread American data on it, yet it is now being launched as a "brand-new drug," although the rest of the world has been growing old on it.

"The thing that irks me," says one drug company spokesman, "is that the thalidomide tragedy has enshrined a bureaucracy. Since 1962 we have been dealing with an agency that has been congratulating itself about its own indecisiveness. It would not be so bad if they could point to thalidomide and say, 'We knew that that drug would be bad for the fetus,' but they didn't know that, they didn't know anything—we averted tragedy through pure dumb lethargy."

Another spokesman who prefers to be nameless likens the FDA to the US Post Office. "It's like arguing that a slowdown in the mail is heroic because there might be a letter bomb with your family's name on it."

Nor can it be argued that in the years since the thalidomide calamity our society has not suffered its share of tragedies. We have had the DES scandal and the more recent Rely tampon problem, so we have not been totally protected.

What we are talking about is a matter of priorities. As I have repeated so often, medicine involves risks. But if fear of those risks is our only criterion, then we will continue to slip into becoming a second-rate research nation.

What with oil crises, dollar crises, export crises, and auto crises, it is not very welcome news that now even America's position in medicine may be eroding. But the sad truth is that this is exactly what is happening, and it is creating a worldwide crisis in research. Here is how it looks to the *British Medical Journal*, one of the more prestigious, and conservative, science publications:

> The delay in introducing new drugs in the United States compared with other countries has become known as the "drug lag." Despite official claims to the contrary, valuable drugs have been partially or wholly denied to the American people for long periods. Critics have argued that the United States Food and Drug Administration has been depriving rather than protecting the public, or even cynically avoiding risk by waiting to see what happens elsewhere. . . .
>
> America is of overriding importance to the pharmaceutical industry. It represents 18 percent of the world drug market and no international manufacturer can afford to ignore it. Yet the Center for the Study of Drug Development has reported that between 1974 and 1976 the number of new chemical entities reaching

Significant Mood Changers Not Available in United States

Drug and manufacturer	Country and date first marketed	History with the FDA	Description
Antidepressants			
mianserin (Organon)	United Kingdom 1976	Research applied for in 1977. Trials still underway.	Tetracyclic antidepressant supposedly safer than tricyclics
nomifensine (Hoechst)	Germany 1976	Research applied for in 1978; now under review.	Belongs to a unique chemical group, may have anticonvulsive properties. Nonsedative and no ill effects on heart.
viloxazine (ICI)	United Kingdom 1974	Research applied for in 1975.	Bicyclic drug (none available in U.S.). May have fewer side effects.
Antipsychotics			
flupenthixol (Lundbeck)	Denmark 1965	Never submitted to FDA by a commercial sponsor.	Long-acting and injectable. In low doses; is an antidepressant

penfluridol (Janssen)	Belgium 1973	Research applied for in 1971. Marketing permit still pending.	Long-acting—can be given once a week. No long-acting antipsychotic now available in US
pimozide (Janssen)	Belgium 1970	Research applied for in 1968, permission to market in 1973. Still pending.	Long-acting—causes less sedation than haloperidol. Used for maintenance therapy in chronic schizophrenia.
pipotiazine (Rhone-Poulenc)	France 1973	Never submitted.	Given only once every 4–6 weeks. Faster onset, less likelihood of depression.
sulpiride (Delagrange)	France 1969	Permission for research has been "pending for 4 to 5 years."	Antipsychotic with anti-depressant qualities. Fewer extrapyramidal effects.

SOURCE: *Medical World News*

NOTE: In fairness to the FDA it should be noted that the "efficacy" of psychotropic drugs is by definition subjective and therefore harder to measure than other forms of medicine. This is one reason why mood-changing drugs are sometimes slower to win approval.

clinical study in the United States fell by nearly half. The few that survive now take about nine more years to reach the market. . . .

If present trends continue, the pharmaceutical industry, which depends heavily on research for its prosperity, seems certain to run down in the coming decade, with serious direct and indirect consequences. Increasing diversification by the big companies already shows their lack of confidence in the future. The trends will be difficult to counteract. Many of the contributory factors are themselves socially desirable, but a growing body of informed opinion holds that the pendulum has swung too far and that the problem must be tackled, whatever the difficulties.*

This shows how our problems are affecting everybody—and nobody worse than the poor third-world countries, where the need for new medicines is so much more obvious.

The life of a US patent on a drug is legally restricted to seventeen years. This period begins with the drug's discovery, or when it is first suspected to have potential benefits. Then the rounds of tests begin, all at the expense of the company that holds the patent. Throughout these tests the "patent clock" is ticking; time is running out on the drug's exclusive ownership.

Thus the delays imposed by regulatory agencies have considerably shortened the effective patent life. In 1966 it was 13.8 years, but by 1977 it had become 8.9 years. Similarly the cost of marketing a new product has risen to an average of more than fifty million dollars. This has placed the drug industry in an unbearable squeeze, with the first area to suffer being basic research.

The pinch on creativity leads to other problems. One is what is sometimes called me-too drug making. This is the practice of spinning off a "new" drug from an older drug that has prior approval. The nature of the FDA is such that it is highly suspicious of anything innovative. It is so suspicious that it routinely disallows any studies based on foreign clinical trials. The result of this

*British Medical Journal 280: 670, 1980.

attitude is that many of the drug companies now place top priority on copycat medicines. Why risk spending years in red tape when you can bring out a drug that acts just like some other drug?

We have Librium, for example, and Valium and Dalmane. We have Sinequan, Serax, Atarax and Trancopal. One might well wonder just how nervous we have become that we need so many products whose effects are so similar!

And yet each of these products, similar as they are, still has to go through the same clinical research, with the same kind of animal trials, the same "double blind" and "cross-over" human studies. This makes for enormous duplication. A sound clinical trial may take years to orchestrate. But when you get all through, perhaps all you have created is an additional burden of statistics and paperwork.

The problem, it would seem—or at least a good part of it—is that bureaucracy values procrastination. Few employees get fired for *not* having done something—and indeed, as we have seen, some can even get medals for it. But against this nightmare of red tape and procrastination, as I make my rounds through the hospital's mental wards, I can't help wondering how many of these patients would be released and free if I had better medicines for them. Who speaks for them? Does anybody care? We have plenty of people who are anxious to "protect" them, but when it comes to healing, everybody fades—it is not a concept that fits well with Big Brotherism.

Here are some parallels: In today's sluggish climate, where the slightest risk has become unacceptable, we would not have been able to achieve approval of lithium, chlorpromazine or reserpine, and we would certainly not have gotten approval for the MAO inhibitors. Since these drugs are potentially dangerous, approval of them would be bogged down in more clinical analysis. Someone, somewhere, would have had bad effects from them, and this would be seen by Washington as a reason to prohibit them. I have heard it said that if aspirin were new, it would take ten years to win its approval. There are people whose stomachs bleed from aspirin, and that would be enough to delay its marketing.

In the case of the sulfa drugs, we lost 106 people on a chemist's misjudgment. Sulfa, being so radical and new, would never get through the present bureaucracy. And yet sulfa, which we had available to us within a year of its discovery, was the greatest lifesaver of the Allied war effort. Offsetting our losses were incalculable gains, but we would not have known them had we been ruled by timidity.

Penicillin—what a dangerous drug this is! There are many people who simply can't tolerate it. Some have died—it can often prove lethal—yet I don't know too many who would wish to get rid of it.

It would probably take penicillin at least twenty years to get approval from our current government. How many people are alive today because penicillin saved them during the 1940s and 1950s?

There is another aspect that also troubles me. Innovative drugs are our tools of research. We would know very little about neurology or brain function were it not for drugs with a built-in risk factor. In the world today there are radically new drugs, but American researchers are virtually ignorant of them. You are probably proud that American hospitals contain the finest hardware and technology available. You have heard this boast from my own profession, particularly when threatened with "socialized medicine." But I am here to tell you that all this wonderful technology—the CAT-scans, PET-scans, the intensive-care life-savers—would have very little value if it weren't for drugs and the avenues of research they have opened up for us.

Paralleling this problem and in some ways complicating it are the tremendously high prices for which drugs are now selling. It is not unusual in some specialties of medicine to pay up to a dollar for one pill or one capsule. As a doctor, I find this an unconscionable burden. How can patients be asked to pay that much? Often these costs are not covered by insurance, particularly when the illness is deemed "psychological."

This, of course, is an issue on which consumerism has focused. Consumerists' primary concern has been the cost of health care. But I fear that sometimes, in their worries about cost, they do not understand all the other variables.

274

Rumor has it that in Washington, D.C., there are two "reforms" now being considered. One would shorten the life of a drug patent; the other would require the pooling of research knowledge. It seems to me that neither of these would be satisfactory—not unless you are willing to go whole hog and eliminate free enterprise from the area of drug making.

The drug makers contend, and perhaps justifiably, that the seventeen-year patent life is already too limited. With half that time spent in FDA paperwork, they have very few years in which to recoup their research expenses. This, of course, helps drive up drug prices. They have to make their profit within a specific time span. After seventeen years, whatever drug they are marketing becomes grist for the mills of the generic drug houses.

"It's worse than that," says one drug-company executive. "Generic drug companies are not that respectful. Often they will go ahead and copy your drug and distribute it even while your patent is valid. They know that bringing them to court is expensive. They hope that you will decide to forego those costs. We don't, of course, because we can't afford to. We take them to court as a matter of principle."

Generic drugs are a boon to consumers, but they are a double-edged sword, and you should know it. Generic drug firms do not do research—they are only in the business of manufacturing. The patented drug is the product of science; the generic drug is only the by-product. It hardly seems fair to pass legislation that would favor the imitator while penalizing the researchers.

The consumer groups say that a shorter patent life might help eliminate duplication. They ask, as I do, why we need so many products whose chemistry and purpose are basically similar. The drug companies argue that this criticism has merit, but that shorter patents are not the solution. They say that the villain is the FDA, which has made "me-too" drugs a business necessity.

As for the pooling of research, while this may be attractive at least from the standpoint of cutting redundancy, it will further discourage innovative science and may well spell the end of the free-enterprise market system in this field.

A great deal depends on how all this is solved: your rights as a

275

patient, and mine as a doctor; the drug companies' right to pursue profit through research, and the government's duty to protect its citizenry. One thing for sure—the problem must be resolved. The whole world is looking to this country for leadership, not only because we are innovators in medicine but because, as consumers, we are a necessary marketplace.

And I, of course, have my own special reasons. As a disciple of Freud from the University of Nebraska, I have been both witness and willing accomplice to one of the greatest revolutions in the history of medicine. I have seen the end of *The Snake Pit* era. I have watched the dismantling of padded cells. I have seen the straitjacket fade into memory along with the white-coated men who administered it. I have watched the healing of agonized victims. I have seen broken families become whole and at peace again. I have seen a profession that was fumbling in subjectivism become a full-fledged member of the community of medicine.

We are fond of saying in psychiatry today that we know about as much as cardiologists. The heart has its secrets, and so does the brain, but we are about equally advanced in our understanding of each. What tomorrow holds I can't say for sure. It is enough for me that there be a tomorrow. But we need the help of an intelligent citizenry. We want to keep going. Are you willing to follow us?

A Selected Bibliography

The serious student of psychiatry and mental illness can do no better than to consult the *Comprehensive Textbook of Psychiatry II*, edited by Alfred M. Freedman, Harold I. Kaplan, and Benjamin J. Sadock (2 vols.), published in Baltimore by Williams & Wilkins (1976).

Other good background sources include *Psychopharmacology: From Theory to Practice*, edited by Jack D. Barchas, Philip A. Berger, Roland D. Ciaranello and Glen R. Elliott, published in New York by Oxford University Press (1977); *Principles of Psychopharmacology*, edited by W. G. Clark and J. del Giudice, published in New York and London by Academic Press (1970); *The Pharmacological Basis of Therapeutics, Fifth Edition*, edited by Louis S. Goodman and Alfred Gilman, published in New York by Macmillan (1980); and *The Harvard Guide to Modern Psychiatry*, edited by Armand M. Nicoli, Jr., published in Cambridge, Mass., and London by Belknap Press of Harvard University Press (1978).

Other works relevant to the material in this book include:
Alpert, Murray, and Arnold J. Freidhoff. "An Un-Dopamine

277

Hypothesis of Schizophrenia." *Schizophrenia Bulletin,* Vol. 6, No. 3. National Institute of Mental Health, 1980.

Balter, Mitchell B., and Jerome Levine. *The Nature and Extent of Psychotropic Drug Usage in the United States.* Presented before the Subcommittee on Monopoly of the Select Committee on Small Business, U.S. Senate. Mimeographed. July 16, 1969.

Balter, Mitchell B., Jerome Levine and Dean I. Manheimer. "Special Article: Cross-National Study of the Extent of Anti-Anxiety/Sedative Drug Use." *New England Journal of Medicine,* Vol. 290, April 4, 1974.

Barbeau, A. "Emerging Treatments: Replacement Therapy with Choline or Lecithin in Neurological Diseases." *Le Journal Canadien des Sciences Neurologiques,* Vol. 5, No. 21, February, 1978.

Barchas, Jack D., Glenn R. Elliott, and Philip A. Berger, Eds. "Biogenic Amine Hypothesis of Schizophrenia." *Psychopharmacology: From Theory to Practice.* New York: Oxford, 1977.

Bauer, William R., F. H. C. Crick, and James H. White. "Supercoiled DNA." *Scientific American,* Vol. 243, No. 1, July, 1980.

Berger, F. M. "Therapeutic Uses of Meprobamate and the Propanediols." *Drug Treatment of Mental Disorders,* edited by Lance L. Simpson. New York: Raven Press, 1976.

Bockar, Joyce A. *Primer for the Nonmedical Psychotherapist.* New York: Spectrum, 1976.

Bookman, Phillip H., and Lowell O. Randall. "Therapeutic Uses of Benzodiazepines." *Drug Treatment of Mental Disorders,* edited by Lance L. Simpson. New York: Raven Press, 1976.

Caldwell, A. "History of Psychopharmacology." *Principles of Psychopharmacology,* edited by W. G. Clark and J. del Guidice, New York and London: Academic Press, 1970.

———*Origins of Psychopharmacology from CPZ to LSD.* Springfield, Ill.: Thomas, 1970.

Clark, Matt, Sharon Begler, and Mary Hager. "The Miracles of Spliced Genes." *Newsweek,* Vol. XCV, No. 11, March 17, 1980.

Cohen, Sidney. "Valium: Its Use and Abuse." *Drug Abuse & Alcoholism Newsletter,* Vol. 5, No. 4, May, 1976.

Cole, Jonathan O. "Phenothiazines." *Drug Treatment of Mental Disorders,* edited by Lance L. Simpson. New York: Raven Press, 1977.

Comptroller General. "Report to the Subcommittee on Science, Research, and Technology, House Committee on Science and Technology: FDA Drug Approval—A Lengthy Process that Delays the Availability of Important New Drugs." United States General Accounting Office. HRD-80-64. May, 28, 1980.

"Drug Lag Bad: Drug Lag Worse." *British Medical Journal,* Vol. 280, No. 670, 1980. Reprinted in *Drug Therapy,* Vol. 10, No. 6, June, 1980.

"Drug Lag '80: The Missing Medicines." *Medical World News,* September 1, 1980.

Faden, Vivian B. "Mental Health: Statistical Note No. 137— Primary Diagnosis of Discharges from Non-Federal General Hospital Psychiatric Inpatient Units, United States, 1975." U.S. Department of Health, Education and Welfare. Mimeographed. August, 1977.

Finkle, Bryan S., Kevin L. McCloskey, and Louis S. Goodman. "Diazepam and Drug-Associated Deaths: A Survey in the United States and Canada." *Journal of the American Medical Association,* Vol. 242, No. 5, August 3, 1979.

Frankel, Glenn. "The Lobotomy Era." *The Washington Post,* April 6, 7, 8, 1980.

Goldsmith, William. *Psychiatric Drugs for the Non-Medical Mental Health Worker.* Springfield, Ill.: Thomas, 1977.

Greengard, Paul. "The Vitamins: Introduction." *The Pharmacological Basis of Therapeutics,* edited by Louis S. Goodman and Alfred Gilman. New York: Macmillan, 1970.

Hixson, Joseph R. "New Hope for Hyperactive Children." *The New York Times Magazine,* August 24, 1980.

Hollister, Leo E. "Antipsychotic Medications and the Treatment of Schizophrenia." *Psychopharmacology From Theory to Practice,* edited by Jack D. Barchas, Philip A. Berger, Roland D.

Ciaranello and Glen R. Elliott. New York: Oxford University Press, 1977.

———"Psychopharmacology in Its Second Generation." *Military Medicine,* Vol. 141, No. 6, June, 1976.

———"Valium: A Discussion of Current Issues." *Psychosomatics,* Vol. 18, January / February / March, 1977.

Iversen, L. L., and A. V. P. MacKay. "Pharmacodynamics of Antidepressants and Antimanic Drugs." *Psychopharmacology of Affective Disorders,* edited by E. S. Paykel and A. Coppen. Oxford, New York, Toronto: Oxford University Press, 1979.

Kety, Seymour S. "Recent Genetic and Biochemical Approaches to Schizophrenia." *Drug Treatment of Mental Disorders,* edited by Lance L. Simpson. New York: Raven Press, 1976.

Kline, Nathan S. *From Sad to Glad: Kline on Depression.* New York: Ballantine, 1974.

Lear, John. *Recombinant DNA: The Untold Story.* New York: Crown, 1978.

Manheimer, Dean I., Susan T. Davidson, Mitchell B. Balter, Glen D. Mellinger, Ira H. Cisin, and Hugh J. Parry. "Popular Attitudes and Beliefs About Tranquilizers." *American Journal of Psychiatry,* Vol. 130, No. 11, November, 1973.

Marks, John. *The Benzodiazepines: Use, Overuse, Misuse, Abuse.* Lancaster, England: MTP Press, 1978.

Mellinger, Glen D., Mitchell B. Balter, Hugh J. Parry, Dean I. Manheimer, and Ira H. Cisin. "An Overview of Psychotherapeutic Drug Use in the United States." *Drug Use: Epidemiological and Sociological Approaches,* edited by Eric Josephsen and Eleanor E. Carroll. Reprint. Hemisphere Publishing, 1974.

Mindham, R. H. S. "Tricyclic Antidepressants and Amine Precursors." *Psychopharmacology of Affective Disorders,* edited by E. S. Paykel and A. Coppen. Oxford, New York, Ontario: Oxford University Press, 1979.

Opler, Marvin K. "Cross-Cultural Uses of Psychoactive Drugs (Ethnopsychopharmacology)." *Principles of Psychopharmacology,* edited by W. G. Clark and J. del Giudice. New York and London: Academic Press, 1970.

Parry, Hugh J. "Use of Psychotropic Drugs by U.S. Adults." *Public Health Reports*, Vol. 83, No. 10, October, 1968.

Pfefferbaum, Adolf. "The Placebo." *Psychopharmacology: From Theory to Practice*, edited by Jack D. Barchas, Philip A. Berger, Roland A. Ciaranello, and Glen R. Elliott. New York: Oxford, 1977.

Pollack, Earl S. "Memorandum #6: Resident Patient Rate in State Hospitals Reduced to One-fourth the 1955 Rate." Alcohol, Drug Abuse and Mental Health Administration, National Institute of Mental Health. Mimeographed. June 27, 1977.

"Psychiatry on the Couch." *Time*, April 2, 1979.

Shapiro, Arthur K., and Louis A. Morris. "The Placebo Effect in Medical and Psychological Therapies." Mimeographed.

Simpson, Lance L., and Bruce Cabot. "Monoamine Oxidase Inhibitors." *Drug Treatment of Mental Disorders*, edited by Lance L. Simpson. New York: Raven Press, 1976.

Tallman, John F., Steven M. Paul, Philip Skolnick, and Dorothy W. Gallagher. "Receptors for the Age of Anxiety: Pharmacology of the Benzodiazepines." *Science*, Vol. 207, January 18, 1980.

Index

Acetylcholine, 78, 163, 164, 166, 175–76
Acute psychosis, diet pills and, 189–90
Adaptive mechanism, 80, 82, 225; flight-or-flight response as, 59, 119
Addiction, 18, 20, 69–70, 188, 235–36; defined, 52; and diet of addicts, 173, 181; and schizophrenia, 141, 142; to Valium, 47–49, 51–54, 122, 210, 211; *See also* Alcoholism
Adenosine triphosphate (ATP), 206
S-Adenosylmethionine, 153
Administrations of drugs, 74–76, 162
Adrenaline, 178, 179, 240
Adrenochrome hypothesis of schizophrenia, 154, 155
Adrenocorticotropic hormone (ACTH), 240–42
Affect: mood synonymous with, 83; of schizophrenics, 140–41, 148
Affective disorders, 82; *See also* Depression
Age: and Gilles de la Tourette's syndrome, 168; and manic-depression, 103; schizophrenia and, 142; *See also* Elderly, the
Agoraphobia, 125, 126
Ailurophobia, 125
Alcohol, 9, 20, 46, 53, 215, 228; for phobias, 127; and schizophrenia, 141, 142; Valium with, 56
Alcoholism: and diet of alcoholics, 172, 181; drug abuse and, 188; as form of self-therapy, 235–36; among men, 100; prevalence of, 210; Valium in treatment of, 55
Allergies, 183
Amniocentesis, 205

Amphetamines, 54, 55, 190, 236, 243; effects of, 145–47, 193; therapeutic value of, 233–34
Anorexia nervosa, 127, 199
Anticholinesterase, 176
Antidepressants: for anxiety, 119; listed by brands, 96; new, 194–96; *See also specific antidepressants*
Antihistamines, 26–29, 163
Antipsychotics, *see specific antipsychotics*
Anxiety, 18, 45–47, 52, 118–24, 181, 193, 210; phobias and, 125–27; symptoms of, 224–25, 228
Anxiety neurosis, 123
Anxious depression, 123
Apomorphine, 146
Artane, 163
Aspirin, 184, 273
Atarax, 273
Autonomic nervous system, 64
Aventyl (nortriptyline), 96
Azathioprine, 215

Barbiturates, 50, 51, 54, 81, 127, 188, 233, 236
Behavior modification, 128–29, 133
Belonophobia, 125–26
Benadryl, 163
Benzedrine, 240
Benzodiazepines, 42, 212; *See also specific drugs*
Biofeedback, 225–32
Bipolar depression, *see* Manic-depression
Blood-brain barrier, 74, 91, 92
Blood busting, 244
Blood-sugar levels: low, 177–81
Blunted affect of schizophrenics, 140–41

282

Body-mind interplay, *see* Mind-body interplay
Brain: cortex of, 64, 68; hemispheres of, 237–38; impulses decoded by, 68; physiology of, 61–64; *See also* Hypothalamus; Limbic system; Neurotransmitters
Butyrophenones, 161–62; *See also specific drugs*

Carbidopa, 76
Castration anxiety, 121
Cells: nerve, 61–65, 68; progenitor, 248–49; ribosomes of cells, 252, 256; structure of 252–53
Central nervous system, 64; *See also* Brain
Childbearing by schizophrenics, 144–45
Chlorpromazine, *see* Thorazine
Chocolate, 181–82
Cholesterol, 175–76
Choline, 174–77
Chromosomes, 253; X-chromosome hypothesis, 99–100, 199
Chronic anxiety, 119
Claustrophobia, 126
Cocaine, 28, 236
Cogentin, 163
Cognitive theory of depression, 84–85
Common signs of schizophrenia, 141–42
Compazine (prochlorperazine), 161
Contraindications: imipramine, 93; lithium, 106; Valium, 55–56
Cortex, 64, 68
Corticosteroids, 97
Cortisol, 97, 98, 105, 241
Cortisone, 242
Counterphobias, 130
CPZ, *see* Thorazine
Creatine, 206
Creatine phosphokinase (CPK), 206–8
Cytoplasm of cell, 252

Dalmane, 37, 273
Darvon, 49
Deaths: attributed to Valium, 48–51; due to sulfa drugs, 264–65; effects of psychoactive drugs on

number of, in hospitals, 21
Deinstitutionalization, 17–18, 21, 30, 31
Dependency, *see* Addiction
Depersonalization neuroses, 123
Depression: 33, 80–101, 188, 225, 236, 250; bipolar (*see* Manic-depression); and blood sugar levels, 179–81; and chocolate consumption, 181, 182, defined, 85–86; due to diet pills, 190; among the elderly, 113–17, 174; female, 106–13; inheritability of, 33, 81, 87, 99–101, 199; neurotransmitters involved in, 66, 74, 88–96, 192–93; new research into, 192–203; predrug approach to, 84–88; role of electrolytes in, 98–99; role of endocrine system in, 97–98; social factors of, 81; types of, 83–84
Desensitization technique, 129
Diabetes: hypoglycemia and, 177
Dialysis schizophrenia, 157–59
Dibenzoxazepines, 161; *See also specific drugs*
Diet: of the elderly, 115–16; Feingold, for hyperactivity, 183–87; *See also* Choline; Food additives and dyes; Food-drug interaction; Lecithin; Tryptophan; Vitamins; *and specific foods*
Diet pills, 189–90
Diethylstilbestrol (DES), 269
DNA (deoxyribonucleic acid), 248–62
L-Dopa, 75, 76, 147, 204
Dopamine, 74, 76, 146, 162–63; effects of diet pills on, 190; effects of food dyes on, 185; in Parkinson's disease, 75, 147; role of, in Gilles de la Tourette's disease, 168; role of, in schizophrenia, 71, 147, 148, 151, 153, 154, 164, 166, 203–4, 207; role of vitamin C in formation of, 173; storage and synthesis of, 240;
Double helix of DNA, 253–54
Drug abuse, *see* Addiction

283

Iatroplacebogenics, 221, 225
Immunoglobulins, 208
Implosion technique, 129, 130
Impulse anxiety, 121
Inappropriate affect in schizo-
    phrenia, 148
Inderal (propranolol), 123–24
Indolones, 161
Indols, 152, 154, 155
Inheritability: of alcoholism, 100; of
    depression, 33, 81, 87, 99–101,
    199; of manic-depression, 103;
    of schizophrenia, 51, 142, 144,
    148–51, 205–7, 209, 257–58
Inhibitory transmitter: GABA as,
    212
Insomnia, 87, 188, 201–2
Institutionalization: effects of drugs
    on, 17–18, 21, 30, 31; for schizo-
    phrenia, 142
Insulin, 178–80
Insulin therapy, 30
Intelligence: chemical improvement
    of, 240–42, 244; of obsessive
    individuals, 132; positron-emis-
    sion tomography to study, of
    gifted individuals, 243
Involutional melancholia, 113

James-Lange hypothesis, 59, 124,
    179–80, 199
Junk foods, 182

Kemadrin, 163
Krebiozen, 220

Laetrile, 173
Lecithin, 166, 174–77
Libido, 121
Librium (chlordiazepoxide; RO-5-
    0690), 21, 37, 41–45, 54, 69,
    120, 133, 273
Limbic system, 59–60, 68, 82, 147,
    148, 180, 240
Lithium carbonate, 10, 35–37, 89,
    99, 166, 258, 273
Lobotomy, 91, 133–35
Lomotil (diphenoxylate), 160, 164–67
Loxitane (loxapine), 161
LSD (lysergic acid diethylamide),
    152, 154, 155
Ludiomil (maprotiline), 96, 195, 204,
    268

Luteal peak of estrogen production,
    112
Luteinizing hormone (LH), 98, 239

Malaria therapy, 133–34
Malnutrition, see Diet
Mania, 102, 176
Manic-depression (bipolar depres-
    sion), 17, 34–37, 102–6, 138, 258
    behavioral manifestations of,
    138, 141; lithium for, 35–37,
    104–6
MAO inhibitors, see Monoamine
    oxidase inhibitors
Marijuana, 235
Marital status: schizophrenia and,
    141, 142
Marplan (isocarboxazid), 96, 108
Megavitamin therapy, 151–57, 219
Melancholia: involutional, 113
Mellaril (thioridazine), 161
Memory: acetylcholine effects on
    loss of, 176; adrenocorticotropic
    hormone effects on, 241; elec-
    troconvulsive therapy and, 92
Men: effects of major tranquilizers
    on sexual activity of, 238–40;
    See also Sex difference
Menopausal depression, 113–14
Mental illness: psychosomatic nature
    of, 76; See also specific illnesses
Mental institutions, see
    Institutionalization
6-Mercaptopurine, 215
Mescaline, 151–55
Methadone, 55
Methylation process, 151, 153, 215
Metrazol (pentylenetetrazol), 212
MHPG (3-methoxy-4-hydrox-
    yphenylglycol), 199–200
Mianserin, 196, 204
Migraine: chocolate and, 181
Miltown (meprobamate), 37–39, 81,
    127
Mind: defined, 225, 229
Mind-body interplay, 21–23; healing
    and, 223
Minimal brain dysfunction: hyperac-
    tivity and, 183
Minor tranquilizers, see specific
    drugs
Moban (molindone), 161
Modulator enzymes, 197, 198

285

Prolixin (fluphenazine), 162
Pseudodementia, 115
Psychiatric ward: first built (1948), 29
Psychiatrists: and prescription of
    minor tranquilizers, 47; public
    view of, 20; reasons for drop in
    number of, 22–23
Psychoactive drugs: early history of,
    17, 21, 26–37; lessening impact
    of, 245–46; negative and posi-
    tive effects of, 17–17; See also
    specific drugs
Psychoanalytic approach, 67, 267; to
    anxiety, 120–21; to depression,
    83–85, 107–8; ECT and, 34;
    limitations of, 23, 31, 230, 245;
    to obsessive-compulsive neu-
    roses, 131; schizophrenia in,
    142, 148
Psychoses: recombinant DNA for,
    260–61; See also specific psychoses
Psychosurgery, 133–36, 142
Purines, 69, 215
Pyramidal tract, 65

Quaaludes, 233

Reactive anxiety, 123
Reactive depression, 83
Receptor sites, 62; blocking effects
    of drugs on, 71–72
    (See also specific drugs)
Reciprocal inhibition technique,
    129, 130
Recombinant DNA, 259–61
Repression (concept), 121
Reserpine (Rawolfia), 31–34, 37, 83,
    94, 159, 166, 191, 193, 273
Reticular activating system, 147, 148
Re-uptake blocking: by tricyclics,
    72–73, 93
Ribosomes of cells, 252, 256
Ritalin, 183
RNA (ribonucleic acid), 256

Schizophrenia, 17, 29, 82, 89, 102,
    123, 137–67, 250, 259; affect in,
    140–41, 148; chocolate consump-
    tion and, 182; common signs of,
    141–42; CPZ for, 142–43,
    146–47, 157–60; defined, 137;
    dialysis theory of, 157–59; etiol-
    ogy of, 145–48; extrapyramidal

effects of CPZ on, 162–64; in-
    heritability of, 51, 142, 144,
    148–51, 205–7, 209, 257–58;
    lithium for, 105; megavitamin
    therapy for, 151–57, 219; new
    research into, 203–9, 243; role
    of dopamine in, 71, 147, 148,
    151, 153, 154, 164, 166, 203–4,
    207; tardive dyskinesia as effect
    of CPZ, 160, 165–67
Sedatives, 28; See also specific drugs
Separation anxiety, 121, 126
Serax, 273
Serentil (mesoridazine), 161
Serotonin (5-hydroxytryptamine),
    66, 72, 73, 78, 115, 187, 195–96,
    200; role of, in depression, 75,
    88–89, 193
Sex difference: and alcoholism, 100;
    in depression, 100, 113; in Gilles
    de la Tourette's disease, 168; in
    hemispheric structure of the
    brain, 237–38; in hyperactivity,
    183; in manic-depression, 103;
    in phobias, 126; in prescriptive-
    drug abuse, 46; in schizo-
    phrenia, 144
Sexual activity: effects of major tran-
    quilizers on male, 238–40
Side effects: of electroconvulsive
    therapy, 91, 92; See also specific
    drugs
Siderodromophobia, 126
Sinequan (doxepin), 273
Sleep-deprivation therapy, 201
Smoking: addiction to, 53
Social control: chemical, 18–19, 240
Social history of schizophrenics, 141,
    142
Socioeconomic factors of schizo-
    phrenia, 143–44
Sodium, 61, 99, 106
Sodium amobarbitol, 228
Somatopsychic (psychosomatic) na-
    ture of mental illness, 76
Somatostatin, 180
Specificity of new drugs, 195
Stagefright, 124
Stelazine (trifluoperazine), 161, 162
Steroids, 97, 240–41, 243
Straightjackets, 91, 276
Street drugs, 54, 76; See also spe-
    cific drugs

287

288